Neurodevelopmental Disorders

Neurodevelopmental Disorders

A Definitive Guide for Educators

Frank E. Vargo

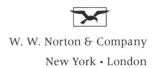

W. W. Norton & Company

New York · London

For information about permission to reproduce selections from this book,
write to Permissions, W. W. Norton & Company, Inc.,
500 Fifth Avenue, New York, NY 10110

For information about special discounts for bulk purchases, please contact
W. W. Norton Special Sales at specialsales@wwnorton.com or 800-233-4830

Manufacturing by Edwards Brothers Malloy
Production manager: Christine Critelli

Library of Congress Cataloging-in-Publication Data
Vargo, Frank E.
Neurodevelopmental disorders : a definitive guide
for educators / Frank E. Vargo. — First edition.
pages cm — (Norton books in education)
Includes bibliographical references and index.
ISBN 978-0-393-70943-8 (hardcover)
1. Children with mental disabilities—Education.
2. Children with autism spectrum disorders—Education.
3. Developmental disabilities. 4. Learning disabilities.
5. Diagnostic and statistical manual of mental disorders. 5th ed.
I. Title.
LC4601.V28 2015
371.9—dc23

2014038404

W. W. Norton & Company, Inc.
500 Fifth Avenue, New York, N.Y. 10110
www.wwnorton.com

W. W. Norton & Company Ltd.
Castle House, 75/76 Wells Street, London W1T 3QT

1 2 3 4 5 6 7 8 9 0

This book is dedicated to my wife,
Cindy Pirro Vargo; my daughter, Erica Vargo;
and all of my cherished family members—
past, present, and future.

Mia famiglia e' tutto per me!

CONTENTS

FIGURES

TABLES

CASE STUDIES

Acknowledgments

I would like to express my sincerest gratitude to all of those who supported me throughout this effort. Many thanks to Deborah Malmud, vice president at W. W. Norton and director of Norton Professional Books. In addition, my thanks to all the professionals at Norton who contributed to and supported this book.

My continued thanks and love also go to my wife, Cindy Pirro Vargo, and our beloved daughter, Erica Vargo. Also, my continual appreciation and affections to Francis and Theresa Vargo, David G. Vargo, Connie Musgrove, Dr. Richard Sprinthall, and Dr. Richard Judah.

Grazie tutto infinite!

Introduction

Neurodevelopmental Disorders: *A Definitive Guide for Educators* provides extensive and practical information to a range of professionals and all others who are interested in the complex and often misunderstood disabilities that fall within the general diagnostic category of neurodevelopmental disorders. This book was purposely written in a format that provides a comprehensive overview of neurodevelopmental deficits and disabilities and related neurocognitive processes, with a strong focus on educational considerations, applications, and relevance across many academic areas. *Neurodevelopmental Disorders* was developed and written with the goal of being a valuable learning tool and resource for educators, clinicians, medical professionals, parents, and all others who may be interested in obtaining initial or additional applied conceptual knowledge in the topic areas (e.g., school and clinical psychologists, counselors, special education professionals, parents of children with special needs, educational adminstrators). The book's writing style is designed to be both practically informative and user friendly for the diverse range of professionals and parents interested in the topic and related considerations, while concurrently remaining well referenced and empirically supported.

Neurodevelopmental Disorders provides a strong focus on understanding current models and theories of neurodevelopmental disorders and related cognitive functions, and the frequent relationships between those topics and many learning disabilities in reading, written language, and mathematics. An overview of specific neurodevelopmental disorders and related clinical syndromes (e.g., attention deficit disorder, autism spectrum disorders, executive function difficulties, language-based learning disabilities, nonverbal learning disability) is also included, with again a strong focus on both applied neurocognitive processes and functions and educational considerations.

A particular focus is the premise that neurodevelopmental functions and disorders occur developmentally, contextually, and uniquely in every human being. Another major theme is the broad and interrelated educational implication(s) and consideration(s) of various neurodevelopmental patterns and profiles, especially involving areas conceptualized and understood as specific learning disabilities.

This book provides readers with valuable and educationally relevant information on a wide range of clinical areas and syndromes classified under the neurodevelopmental disorders. I begin with an overview of current topics and models of neurodevelopmental functions, with a focus on recent research on educationally based neurocognitive development and processes. Next I provide a foundational understanding of the relationships between neurodevelopmental and neurocognitive delays and deficits and the following:

- Many types of language-based learning disabilities
- Many disorders and types of reading disabilities (e.g., various subtypes of developmental dyslexia)
- Many types of written language disabilities (e.g., various subtypes of developmental dysgraphia)
- Many types of math disabilities (e.g., various subtypes of developmental dyscalculia)

- Related clinical syndromes, including attention-deficit/hyper-activity disorder, autism spectrum disorder, and executive function difficulties

This book is the result of many years of integrated clinical practice and applied scholarly research. Thus, the clinical and educational information is integrated with case studies and vignettes to provide readers with contextual examples and illustrations, especially involving many educational considerations and problems.

CHAPTER OUTLINES

Chapter 1 provides an overview of newly organized definitions and criteria of neurodevelopmental disorders, in a less clinically oriented format that will be enjoyably informative to readers across all professional disciplines and other interested individuals. Topics include:

A Definition of Neurodevelopmental Disorders
Types of Neurodevelopmental Disorders
The Value of Diagnostic Labels and Categories
Descriptive Overviews of the Neurodevelopmental Disorders:
Intellectual Disabilities
Communication and Language Disorders
Specific Learning Disorders
Autism Spectrum Disorder
Attention-Deficit/Hyperactivity Disorder
Neurodevelopmental Motor Disorders
Differential Diagnosis

Chapter 2 provides a broad foundation of knowledge regarding the areas of neurodevelopmental constructs and learning. These constructs are organized as both clusters and specific areas of cognitive functions related to areas of neurodevelopmental processes. Topics include definitions and conceptual information on:

The Complexity of Neurodevelopmental Processes
Neurodevelopmental Constructs
  The Concept of Intelligence
  Attention
  Language
  Memory
  Temporal-Sequential Ordering
  Spatial Ordering
  Neuromotor Functions
  Social Cognition
  Higher-Order Cognition

Chapter 3 provides a foundation of knowledge regarding the areas of neurodevelopmental disorders defined as intellectual disabilities. The specific chapter topics include:

Intellectual Disability
Adaptive Behaviors
  Is Intellectual Developmental Disorder the Same as Mental Retardation?
Educational Considerations in Individuals with Intellectual Developmental Disorder
Historical and Developing Concepts of Intelligence
  Crystallized Intelligence and Fluid Intelligence

Chapter 4 describes communication disorders and language disabilities. Illustrative vignettes and case examples help to clarify conceptual understanding. The specific chapter topics include:

Language-Based Neurodevelopmental Disabilities
Common Characteristics of Children With Language and Communication Disorders

Language Disabilities and Psychological and Behavioral
    Disorders
The Five Major Language Components
    Phonology
    Morphology
    Syntax
    Semantics
    Pragmatic Language

Chapter 5 provides a comprehensive overview of the neuro-developmental disorders defined as attention-deficit/hyperactivity disorder. The chapter is rich with case studies and examples to help readers better understand this often misunderstood clinical syndrome and to enhance understanding of the currently understood variations of this disorder. Chapter 5 also covers the topic of neurodevelopmental processes and executive functions. Specific topics include:

Signs and Symptoms of ADHD
The Attention Control System
    Mental Energy Controls
    Processing Controls
    Production Controls
ADHD and Executive Functions
    Executive Functions Defined
    Specific Observable Symptoms and Traits of Poor Executive
    Functioning
    Developmental Considerations
    Neurodevelopmental Considerations

Chapter 6 discusses autism spectrum disorder, including clinical descriptions, diagnostic criteria, and relevant case study analysis. The chapter includes extensive information regarding educational considerations and implications of autism.

Communication Problems Associated With Autism Spectrum Disorder

Restricted or Repetitive Patterns of Behaviors, Activities, or Interests

Conditions That May Coexist With Autism Spectrum Disorder

Educational Considerations

Asperger's Disorder

Symptoms of Asperger's Disorder

Educational Implications

Chapter 7 discusses motor disorders. The specific chapter topics include:

Developmental Coordination Disorder

Dyspraxia

What Is Praxis?

Stereotypic Movement Disorder

Tic Disorders

Tourette Syndrome

Persistent Motor or Vocal Tic Disorder

Provisional Tic Disorder

Chapter 8 discusses a wide range of material regarding specific learning disorders. It clarifies definitions and foundational concepts regarding learning disabilities and provides a framework on extended related topic information presented in chapters 9, 10, and 11. Specific topics include:

Definitions of Learning Disabilities

Signs of Learning Disabilities

Chapter 9 is a comprehensive presentation on neurodevelopmental processes and reading disabilities, including extensive illustrative vignettes and case presentations. Topics include:

Reading and Phonological Processing
    Phonemes and Phonological Awareness
Phonological Memory and the Role of Memory Functions
Implications for Remedial Interventions for Phonological
    Problems
Reading and Word Automaticity
    Word Identification in the Reading Process
    Rapid Naming and Word Retrieval
Other Contributing Factors in Reading Dysfluency
Reading Fluency and Comprehension
    Remedial Interventions for Reading Dysfluency
    Implications for Remedial Interventions
Reading Disorders and Comprehension Deficits
Understanding and Identifying Language Processing
    Disabilities
The Definition of Language and the Five Major Language
    Components
Other Neurodevelopmental Factors That Could Affect Read-
    ing Comprehension
Enhancing Reading Comprehension Abilities in Classrooms

Chapter 10 describes neurodevelopmental processes and disorders of written language. Extensive illustrative vignettes and
case presentations help illustrate the following topic areas:

Processes That Can Inhibit Writing Development
    Attention Deficits and Disorders
    Language Deficits and Disorders
    Memory Deficits and Disorders
    Temporal-Sequential Ordering Deficits and Disorders
    Spatial Ordering Deficits and Disorders
    Neuromotor Deficits and Disorders
    Higher-Order Cognition/Language Deficits and Disorders
    Executive Function Deficits and Disorders

Chapter 11 focuses on neurodevelopmental processes and math disabilities and is also rich in supportive examples and case studies to help present the following topic areas:

Warning Signs of Math Disabilities
Neurodevelopmental Functions and Math Learning Disorders
    Attention Deficits
    Language Deficits
    Memory Deficits
    Temporal-Sequential Ordering Deficits
    Spatial Ordering Deficits
    Neuromotor Deficits
    Higher-Order Cognition and Language Deficits
    Executive Function Deficits

Neurodevelopmental
Disorders

Chapter 1

PRIMARY CONCEPTS OF NEURODEVELOPMENTAL AND NEUROCOGNITIVE PROCESSES

We can think of ourselves, and quite rightly, as information-processing organisms. As you read this page, you are processing information on many levels, and much of those functions and processes are occurring below the threshold of conscious awareness. Consider that while you are reading this page, utilizing multiple and interrelated cognitive processes (that is, processes that involve the brain, such as thinking and reasoning, and many levels of language processing), you are also processing many other types and levels of information. How cold or warm are you? How comfortable is the chair you are sitting on? What other sounds and smells are your senses attuned to? Just as important, how much of that information are you screening out and so consciously unaware of? What are you able to consistently attend to? We are also, then, processing and screening information in and out through many sensory systems that interactively involve the brain, the central nervous system, and related physical senses (Kalat, 2004; Kolb & Wishaw, 2009; Shaffer & Kipp, 2009).

In addition to constantly processing information in multiple ways, we are also dynamic beings that are in a constant state of changing and development, on virtually all levels of human functioning and experience. Those developmental processes, well studied and researched for many years in the developmental sciences, begin prenatally and continue to the end of our lives (Goswami, 2008; Meece & Daniels, 2008; Pressley & McCormick, 2007). The processes of human development do not happen in a biological vacuum but in fact occur within the contexts of interactive and interrelational biological, genetic, environmental, and social functions and experiences that result in constant cognitive and related developmental growth and changes unique to every individual.

A DEFINITION OF NEURODEVELOPMENTAL DISORDERS

The primary focus of this book, in developmental contexts, is neurodevelopment—more specifically, atypical neurodevelopmental processes and functions, which can result in a range of specifically identified neurodevelopmental disorders. Such disorders have been categorized and recognized over past years within the contexts of various clinical and medical models and syndromes (Baty, Carey, & McMahon, 2011; Reynolds & Mayfield, 2011; Teeter & Semrud-Clikeman, 2007).

Cognitive-related disorders (e.g., involving functions of the brain) that are ultimately due to genetic causes and that are present from early childhood are known as neurodevelopmental disorders (Frith, 2008). These disorders can also be understood as a group of conditions that typically have their onset in various developmental periods, most often in early childhood (American Psychiatric Association, 2013; Goldstein & Reynolds, 2011; Yeates, Ris, Taylor, & Pennington, 2010). In physical and more medically understood terms, neurodevelopmental disorders can be characterized as impairments of the brain and central nervous system. From a psychological perspective, neurodevelopmental disorders are commonly defined as conditions of abnormal brain function that typically adversely affect a child's emotional and social functioning and cognitive and learning capabilities over time and across developmental stages (Teeter & Semrud-Clikeman, 2007; Farran & Karmiloff-Smith, 2012; Garralda & Raynaud, 2012; Goldstein & Reynolds, 2011; Goswami, 2008). It is also important to note that neurodevelopmental disorders are innate to an individual. Such disorders can be thought of as the hard wiring of the brain and central nervous system that an individual is born with (Baty et al., 2011; Bauman & Kemper, 1994; Garralda & Raynaud, 2012; Goldstein & Reynolds, 2011).

The causes of various neurodevelopmental disorders include genetic influences, disorders of the immune system, infectious diseases and bacterial infections, nutritional deficiencies, exposure to toxins, physical trauma, medications that may be adverse to a particular individual, and even severe emotional deprivation. A primary consideration in all of these causes includes the specific developmental stage of the individual (including physical and cognitive stages of development) when the variable or event occurred (Baty et al., 2011; Goldstein & Reynolds, 2011; Odom, Horner, Snell, & Blacher, 2007; Reynolds & Mayfield, 2011).

TYPES OF NEURODEVELOPMENTAL DISORDERS

Over time, many disorders with various etiologies have been recognized or classified as neurodevelopmental in nature (Baty et al., 2011; Goldstein & Reynolds, 2011; Yeates et al., 2010). Clinical syndromes and disabilities that are most currently and consistently included under the category of neurodevelopmental disorders include intellectual disabilities, communication and language disorders, specific learning disorders (reading, written language, and mathematics), autism spectrum disorder (ASD), attention-deficit/hyperactivity disorder (ADHD) and related executive function deficits, nonverbal learning disability, and motor disorders and developmental coordination disorder (American Psychiatric Association; 2013; Barnes, Fuchs, & Ewing-Cobbs, 2010; Mervis & John, 2010; Ozonoff, 2010; Pennington, 2009; Peterson & Pennington, 2010; Snowling & Hayiou-Thomas, 2010; Yeates et al., 2010).

THE VALUE OF DIAGNOSTIC LABELS AND CATEGORIES

What is a diagnosis? Is a specific diagnosis of a disorder or disability helpful, or potentially confusing and even potentially problematic to an individual or professionals dealing with such issues? While these questions and other related issues may be worthy of healthy and important discussions and debates, the fact is that diagnostic categories and labels are an important component of most medical, clinical, and educational systems (Batshaw, 1997; Vargo, 2007; Vargo, Young, & Judah, 2008).

While some individuals and professionals across clinical and educational disciplines may argue against the use of labels to describe many syndromes and disabilities, strong arguments can also be made in favor of the value of diagnostic labels and categories across not only medical contexts, but also in regard to clinical and educational situations and models of service and delivery. Some of those considerations of the positive value of diagnostically categorizing disabilities and disorders could include the following:

1. A specific diagnosis enables a range of professionals from different disciplines to organize and identify multiple variables that are common to a specific syndrome or disorder, thus enabling professionals to more effectively identify a particular disorder or disability.
2. A specific diagnosis enables professionals from different disciplines to differentially diagnose disabilities and dis-

orders, and can provide consistent guidelines to professionals to better clarify and more accurately identify a possible alternate medical, clinical, or educational syndrome or disability.

3. A specific diagnosis that involves established criteria agreed upon between different professions and models can provide a solid reference point to more accurately and consistently identify disorders, syndromes, and disabilities. For instance, when an individual is described or previously diagnosed with ASD, virtually all cross-disciplinary professionals (as well as nonprofessionals) involved with that person will have an immediate point of reference and subsequent general understanding of that individual's general issues and clinical and educational profile. A diagnostic system (in many professional models and contexts) can therefore provide a more accurate and valuable framework for communication among all individuals (professionals and otherwise) who need to accurately understand and address a disorder or disability.

4. A specific diagnosis can provide a more accurate and consistent framework to more effectively guide the development and implementation of appropriate and most effective interventions and accommodations for a disorder, based on sound research and established practice treatments and models.

DESCRIPTIVE OVERVIEWS OF NEURODEVELOPMENTAL DISORDERS

Intellectual Disabilities

Intellectual disabilities can be understood as deficits in general mental abilities—more specifically, deficiencies in cognitive areas involving reasoning, abstract thinking, judgment, problem solving, academic functioning, and even one's ability to learn and intellectually grow through experience (Mervis & John, 2010; Pennington, 2009; Rondal, Hodapp, Soresi, Dykens, & Nota, 2004; Yeates et al., 2010). An important component of an intellectual disabilities diagnosis is an impairment in general adaptive functioning, such as a developmentally appropriate ability to manage self-care and safety habits (American Psychiatric Association, 2013; Batshaw, 1997). For older individuals with clinical profiles of primary intellectual deficiencies, deficits in adaptive functioning typically also include significant difficulties in areas involving social and interpersonal functioning, occupational functioning, and independence in living and related life skills (Hassiotis, Barron, & Hall, 2010; Whitaker, 2013).

Communication and Language Disorders

Communication and language disorders include a range of language and related cognitive deficits that may include the form of language (phonology, syntax, morphology), the content of language (semantics), and the function (pragmatics) of language (Catts & Kamhi, 1999; Hanson & Rogers, 2012; Kamhi & Catts, 1989; Quinn, 2010; Vargo, 2007, 2008). Children with language disorders, across all variations and levels of severity, typically share four common symptoms: (1) a deficiency or developmental delay in the quality of language that is learned, comprehended, and produced; (2) deficiencies in grammar understanding and applied usage; (3) developmentally delayed social communication skills; and (4) deficient nonverbal communication skills (Catts & Kamhi, 1999; Hanson & Rogers, 2012; Kamhi & Catts, 1989).

Specific Learning Disorders

The specific learning disorders involve particular deficits in an individual's ability to perceive or process information effectively and subsequent related developmental delays in various areas of specific academic skills sets and abilities (D'Amato, Fletcher-Janzen, & Reynolds, 2005; Fletcher, Lyon, Fuchs, & Barnes, 2007; Levine, 2002; Miller, 2010; Odom et al., 2007; Pennington, 2009). Those academic delays include deficits in various areas of reading, written language, and mathematics (Cimera, 2007; D'Amato et al., 2005; Fletcher et al., 2007). A diagnosis of specific learning disorders assumes or is based on documentation of underlying neurodevelopmental and related neurocognitive deficits that underlie a recognized academic delay and difficulties (American Psychiatric Association, 2013; Miller, 2010; Sadock & Sadock, 2003).

Autism Spectrum Disorder

ASD is a complex neurodevelopmental disorder that is estimated to occur today in approximately 1 out of 150 children, is four times more common in males, and has strong genetic components (American Psychiatric Association, 2013; Bauman & Kemper, 1994; Lang, 2010; Ozonoff, 2010; Pennington, 2009). While ASD occurs across a spectrum of degrees and variations of clinical profiles, three core deficits in functioning and developmental processes are common to the disorder: (1) deficiencies in social interactions and functioning based on expected typical developmental levels, (2) deficits and developmental delays in functional language and communication skills, and (3) restricted areas of personal interest and often observable patterns of stereotypical behaviors (Frith, 2008; Hanson & Rogers, 2012; Rogers, Ozonoff, & Hansen, 2013). While severity and symptomatic patterns of ASD are quite variable, the interrelated symptoms of the disorder will always have a significant effect on an individual's performance and functioning across all areas of living and personal functioning (Frith, 2008; Lang, 2010).

Attention-Deficit/Hyperactivity Disorder

ADHD is a neurodevelopmental disability that occurs across cultures in about 5% of children and about 2.5% of adults

(American Psychiatric Association, 2013). The primary difficulty and diagnostic component evident in children and adults
with ADHD is significant problems regulating and maintaining
attention and focus at developmentally appropriate levels (Barkley, 1997, 1998; Pennington, 2009). The syndrome of ADHD
also typically includes a range of cognitive and processing deficits (Barkley, 1997; Levine, 1995).

It is also now well documented that ADHD typically includes
varying degrees of difficulty in areas categorized as executive
functions. The executive functions are cognitive capabilities
that are mediated primarily through the frontal lobes of the
brain and directly involve a range of specific neurodevelopmental processes (Barkley, 1997; Dawson & Guare, 2004; Goldberg,
2001; Meltzer, 2007; Weyandt, 2005; Willcutt, 2010). Students
with executive function deficits typically have neurobiologically based problems that can particularly affect learning processes involving planning, mental flexibility, organization, and
self-monitoring (Barkley, 1997; Levine, 1995; Meltzer & Krishnan, 2007). Recent and ongoing research has provided strong
and consistent evidence that ADHD is a neurodevelopmental
disorder that results from neurobiological and neurophysiological factors and dysfunctions (Castellanos et al., 2002; Hale et al.,
2010; Miller, 2010a; Pennington, 2009).

Neurodevelopmental Motor Disorders

Neurodevelopmental disorders also include a range of disabilities and developmental delays recognized under the diagnostic category of motor disorders (American Psychiatric
Association, 2013; Donald & Shah, 2013; Sadock & Sadock,
2003; Sugden & Chambers, 2005). The motor disorders in general may involve developmental delays and deficits involving
fine and gross motor functions, which are typically recognized
and understood within various diagnostic models that include

developmental coordination disorder, dyspraxia, childhood apraxia, specific developmental disorder of motor function, developmental coordination disorder, and clumsy child syndrome (American Psychiatric Association, 2013; Ball, 2002; Boon, 2010; Drew & Creek, 2005; Kirby & Drew, 2003; Kurtz, 2007; Pennington, 2009; Woods & Miltenberger, 2009). The movement-related disorders often are also concurrent with a diverse range of learning disabilities and information-processing deficits in children and adults (Jones, 2005; Ripley, 2001; Yeo, 2005).

Developmental coordination disorder has been recognized and described under various labels for at least the past 100 years, with previous diagnostic labels including "motoric deficiency," "minimal brain dysfunction," and "congenital maladroitness" (Ball, 2002; Drew & Creek, 2005; Kirby & Drew, 2003; Sugden & Chambers, 2005; Pennington, 2009; Sadock & Sadock, 2003; Tupper & Sondell, 2004).

Other neurodevelopmental movement disorders include stereotypic movement disorder and tic disorder (American Psychiatric Association, 2013; Donald & Shah, 2013; Walsh, de Bie, & Fox, 2013; Woods & Miltenberger, 2009). A typical clinical profile of stereotypic movement disorders includes patterns of repetitive and seemingly driven yet apparently purposeless motor behaviors. Examples of such repetitive behaviors include movements of the head, body, and hands that are developmentally atypical for a child or adult. Tic disorders involve sudden, rapid, and recurrent nonrythmic motor movements or vocalizations. Such motoric or vocal manifestations are observably involuntary in an individual diagnosed with tic disorder, although the episodes can often be voluntarily controlled for short periods of time (Drew & Creek, 2005; Kirby & Drew, 2003; Sugden & Chambers, 2005; Woods & Miltenberger, 2009).

DIFFERENTIAL DIAGNOSIS

It is clear from clinical research and practice that diagnostic profiles and symptoms can overlap in various neurodevelopmental diagnostic categories (American Psychiatric Association, 2013; Ball, 2002; Jones, 2005; Kurtz, 2007; Ripley, 2001). For instance, an individual with a primary diagnosis of ASD may exhibit unique patterns of stereotypical motor or vocal behaviors (Frith, 2008; Hanson & Rogers, 2012; Lang, 2010; Ozonoff & Hansen, 2013; Rogers & Ozonoff, 2010; Rogers et al., 2013), and a child or adult with a primary diagnosis of intellectual disability may subsequently present with developmental delays in various facets of language function and understanding, as well as developmental deficits in social functioning and awareness (Hassiotis et al., 2010; Mervis & John, 2010; Pennington, 2009; Rondal et al., 2004; Yeates et al., 2010; Whitaker, 2013). An individual with a primary diagnosis of nonverbal learning disability may also have quite significant problems with various areas of motor coordination and visual-spatial information processing (Palombo, 2006; Rourke, 1989, 1995b). Since overlaps in cognitive dysfunction, clinical symptomology, and developmentally atypical behavioral and vocal patterns commonly occur between and within various neurodevelopmental syndromes and clinical profiles, it would seem imperative that effective diagnostic procedures be utilized to maximize the accuracy and clinical identification of a potential primary neurodevelopmental disorder.

Chapter 2

NEURODEVELOPMENTAL CONSTRUCTS AND LEARNING

This chapter outlines a broad foundation of knowledge regarding the areas of neurodevelopmental constructs and related learning processes. The neurodevelopmental constructs are organized as both clusters and specific areas of cognitive functions related to areas of neurodevelopmental processes. The chapter includes definitions and conceptual information on the following topics:

General intelligence
Crystallized intelligence
Fluid intelligence
Attention
Language
Memory
Spatial ordering
Temporal-sequential ordering
Neuromotor functions
Social cognition
Higher-order cognition
Executive functions

Neurodevelopmental constructs can be thought of as neuro-cognitive processes that interactively facilitate virtually all aspects of learning and cognitive functioning. A neurodevelopmental function may be quite specific, such as an aspect of a memory process (Lezak, Howieson, & Loring, 2004; Lyon & Krasnegor, 1996). A neurodevelopmental process may also be very complex, such as the various integrated cognitive components involved in attention regulation (Barkley, 1997, 1998). Deficits in underlying neurophysiological and related neurodevelopmental processes that facilitate learning and cognitive functions can manifest in a very wide range of difficulties for an individual, which can be observed in such domains as academic, vocational, and social functioning (Levine, 2002; Kibby, 2009).

THE COMPLEXITY OF NEURODEVELOPMENTAL PROCESSES

If you put your two closed fists together with fingers touching, you will have the approximate size of your brain, the source of all cognitive functions and the biological center of yourself. While relatively small in size and perhaps visually unassuming, the human brain is currently the most complex system that we are currently aware of in the universe (Carter, 2009). It may be easy to conceptualize the brain as a single unit, but in truth it is composed of trillions of individual cells that are constantly communicating with each other through complex and interactive biochemical and electrical processes (Carter, 2009; Kalat, 2004; Nolte, 2009; Ornstein & Thompson, 1984). The individual communicating cells of the brain create a webbing network of connections, or synapses. The number of such potential synaptic connections in one human brain has been estimated to be as high as 30 trillion (Carter, 2009; Kalat, 2004; Kandel, Schwartz, & Jessell, 2000). The sheer and almost unimaginable volume and possibilities of connections in the brain allow for a virtually endless combination of neurodevelopmental events and related cognitive functions (Berninger & Richards, 2002; Kandel et al., 2000; Levine, 2002).

NEURODEVELOPMENTAL CONSTRUCTS

As many as 15–30% of children may suffer school failures because of learning disorders that result from subtle deficiencies in neurological development or mild brain dysfunctions (Levine, 1995). In most cases the causes of neurodevelopmental disorders are unknown, although genetic contributions, chromosomal disorders, birth complications, head injury, and prenatal maternal alcohol or drug abuse may be underlying factors in many such conditions. Medication may temporarily disguise neurodevelopmental problems, and standardized tests of cognitive functions may not detect many of the common and serious dysfunctions (Levine, 1995). Mental health professionals might consider a child's neurodevelopmental status before undertaking clinical interventions such as individual and family counseling (Vargo, 2008).

While the number of combinations of potential neurodevelopmental connections and resulting cognitive function outcomes cannot even be estimated, there are models of neurodevelopmentally based constructs that cluster into general cognitive areas and subareas. Pennington (2009) outlined a model of psychometric constructs based on the earlier theories of Cattell and Horn (1978) that included the constructs of general intelligence, crystallized intelligence, and fluid intelligence. That model also included other interrelated cognitive components involving working memory functions and speed of information processing. Pennington (2009) also emphasized the importance of neurodevelopmental constructs in learning that include various areas of language, multiple components of visual perception, types of memory processes, executive functions, and social cognition and awareness.

Levine (2002) posited a model of neurodevelopmental systems that has eight general components that are interrelated and dependent on each other in all cognitive and related activities. The eight components include:

1. The attentional control system
2. The memory system
3. The language system
4. The spatial ordering system
5. The sequential ordering system
6. The motor system
7. The higher thinking system
8. The social thinking system

Over the past several decades, additional models of human cognitive functioning have emerged, based on previous theories as well as the integration of ongoing research in the neurosciences, cognitive psychology, the developmental sciences, and related educational disciplines (Goswami, 2008; Sattler, 2001; Sprinthall & Sprinthall, 1999). In 1997, American psychologist John Carroll proposed a factor-analytic theory of cognitive abilities, composed of three general strata or levels (Carroll, 1997; Flanagan, Genshaft, & Harrison, 1997; Sattler, 2001). Within the context of the three general strata posited by Carroll, other cognitive factors comprising intelligence and cognition were included, such as information retrieval capacities and a more diverse range of memory systems and functions. Carroll's model also emphasized more extensive subcomponents of neurodevelopmental processes within the more general cognitive clusters.

Other more contemporary cognitive models include an information-processing theory of intelligence that integrates other cognitive factors into the learning process, such as newly researched areas of metacognition, schematic knowledge, cognitive control processes, and the cognitive executive system (Borkowski, 1985; Campione & Brown, 1978; Reynolds & French, 2005; Sattler, 2001). Another theory of human intelligence was proposed by American psychologist and psychometrician Robert Sternberg, who emphasized a triarchic division of general cognitive dimensions involving a component dimension, an experiential dimension, and a contextual dimension of intelligence (Sattler, 2001; Sternberg, 1986). Sternberg's triarchic theory of intelligence also included a number of interactive cognitive subcomponents involving higher-order thinking and reasoning, active task execution strategies, automatization of mental processes, and environmental adaptation capabilities.

As research on cognitive abilities involving multiple areas of human information processing progressed, further models of human cognition and intelligence emerged. One such model involved the integration of planning processes, attentional processes, and simultaneous and sequential processing abilities (Dass, Naglieri, & Kirby, 1994). Also known as PASS (planning-attention-simultaneous-successive processing), that proposed model of human cognition was influenced by earlier pivotal research by neuropsychologist Aleksandr Luria (1966a, 1966b).

The Concept of Intelligence

Definitions of intelligence across most current relevant theories and models of cognition include attributes such as basic mental processes, adaptation to the environment, processes of higher-order thinking (e.g., reasoning, problem solving, and decision making), and the ability to learn and effectively apply abstract thinking skills and logic (Pennington, 2009; Sattler, 2001; Sprinthall & Sprinthall, 1990; Sternberg & Berg, 1986; Terman, 1921; Wechsler, 1958, 2001, 2002).

Some major theories of intelligence emphasize a more pragmatic applied view of intellectual processes, stating that intelligence can be recognized by what it enables us to do (Sattler, 2001; Wechsler, 1958, 2001, 2002). Another important model posits a theory of multiple intelligences (Gardner, 1983). Gardner's model, in addition to including components of intellectual cognition that involve linguistic and spatial understanding and applications, also includes other specific areas of intelligence, including logical-mathematical intelligence, body-kinesthetic intelligence, musical intelligence, and various subtypes of personal intelligence.

While there are obviously many ways and theories to define intelligence, experts in the fields of psychology, education, genetics, biology, and sociology generally agree that the important elements of intelligence include the following constructs and applied abilities (Cattell, 1943; Gardner, 1983; Ginsburg & Opper, 1987; Gruber & Voneche, 1995; Meece & Daniels, 2008; Piaget, 1972; Lezak et al., 2004; Pressley & McCormick, 2007; Sattler, 2001; Sprinthall & Sprinthall, 1990; Sternberg & Berg, 1986; Terman, 1921; Wechsler, 1958, 2001, 2002):

1. Abstract reasoning or thinking capabilities
2. The ability to solve problems through applied reasoning processes
3. Linguistic competence and related reasoning and understanding capacities
4. Visual-spatial processing and reasoning
5. Applied multiple functions of memory
6. Speed and efficiency of mental processing
7. The capacity to acquire knowledge
8. A fund of acquired general knowledge
9. Mathematical competence
10. Adaptation to one's environment
11. Applied creativity

Attention

Ongoing research has clearly provided strong and consistent evidence that ADHD is a neurodevelopmental disorder that results from neurobiological and neurophysiological factors and dysfunctions (Castellanos et al., 2002; Hale et al., 2010; Miller, 2010a; Pennington, 2009). The primary difficulty and diagnostic component evident in children and adults with ADHD is significant problems regulating and maintaining attention and focus at developmentally appropriate levels (Barkley, 1997, 1998; Pennington, 2009). What may be less commonly understood about ADHD is that the disorder typically manifests in cognitive-related dysfunctions involving mental energy, processing controls, and production control (Levine, 1995), as well as the ability to follow through and finish tasks, problems with impulse control, and difficulties mediating selective attention processes (Barkley, 1997; Levine, 2002).

The syndrome of ADHD also typically includes varying degrees of difficulty in areas categorized under the term "executive functions," which are cognitive processes that are mediated primarily through the frontal lobes of the brain and directly involve a range of specific neurodevelopmental processes (Barkley, 1997; Dawson & Guare, 2004; Goldberg, 2001; Meltzer, 2007; Weyandt, 2005; Willcutt, 2010). As such, individuals with ADHD and related executive function deficits typically have neurobiologically based problems that can particularly affect learning processes involving planning, mental flexibility, organization, and self-monitoring of one's learning processes (Barkley, 1997; Levine, 1995; Meltzer & Krishnan, 2007). As previously discussed in this chapter, various cognitive aspects of attention have also been regarded as very important components of general and applied intelligence (Dass et al., 1994; Luria, 1966a, 1966b).

Language

Language problems may occur at many levels of verbal, reading, and writing processing and production. For instance, some students may have difficulties interpreting and manipulating the sounds of language. Learners with language processing difficulties may often overrely on contextual cues to understand linguistic meaning while reading or listening to spoken language. Other language-impaired learners may have difficulties at the semantic level, and subsequently confuse the meanings of words and the relationships among them. Other language-impaired students may confuse syntax, word order, or grammatical forms in written language (Catts, 1996; Catts & Kamhi, 1999; Feifer & DeFina, 2000, 2002; Levine, 1995; Shaywitz, 2003; Singer, 1990). Some specific language-related inabilities related to understanding more abstract and symbolic language concepts are also components of language-based learning disabilities (Catts & Kamhi, 1999).

The ability to understand and articulate language at various developmental levels is a critical component of learning and academic success. It is generally agreed that there are five rule-based parameters of language: (1) phonology, (2) morphology, (3) syntax, (4) semantics, and (5) pragmatics (Catts & Kamhi, 1999; Vargo et al., 2008).

Phonology, which includes cognitive functions understood as general phonological processing, refers to an individual's overall innate ability to hear, discriminate, recognize, and understand the various sound components in language (Vargo et al., 2008; Feifer & DeFina, 2000). Phonological awareness, the ability to hear and understand the sound-symbol correspondences of the printed page, is a critical component of early reading development (Rayner & Pollatsek, 1989). In fact, primary reading skills are facilitated by two primary cognitive functions: phonological processing, which supports reading decoding skills, and word automaticity capacities, which support the automatic and instantaneous retrieval and identification of the visual codes of words (Sanders, 2001; Vargo et al., 2008; Wolf, 2001).

Morphology can be thought of as the study of words and how they are formed. While those interesting letter combinations can be translated from basic phonological components into decoded letter and sound combinations, what is also necessary for letter-sound combinations to make sense in a language is a set of morphological rules that govern how words are made. The related language component that governs those rules is known as morphology (Kuder, 2003; Stacey, 2003).

Syntax can be understood as language at the sentence level. The established rules of syntax govern sentence organization, word order, and the relationship between words. Syntax regulates how words are combined into larger meaningful units of phrases and sentences. Grammatical structures such as noun and verb phrases are also included in syntactical processes (Akmajian, Demers, & Harnish, 1988). Syntax plays a critical role in the understanding and interpretation of grammar and subsequent language meaning (Rayner & Pollatsek, 1989; Singer, 1990).

Semantics is the aspect of language that governs the meanings of words and word combinations (Kuder, 2003; Rayner & Pollatsek, 1989; Singer, 1990). The English language, like many others, is rich with words that have multiple meanings, shades of meaning, and contextually driven meanings. For instance, the word "saw" can be both a noun or a verb, depending on the context of the sentence construct utilized. The ability to understand the rich and diverse meanings of a continually expanding vocabulary base is essential to academic success as a student progresses through educational grade levels. Exposure to high numbers of vocabulary words and concepts begins in the early grade school years, peaks again during the high school years, and continues at the college level (Levine, 2002; Singer, 1990).

Pragmatics involves the use of language in social and environmental contexts. Individuals who are listening to spoken language, engaged in conversation, or reading who are not readily familiar with sociocultural references relative to those processes will simply not have an effective reference point to fill in the meanings that are not literally stated. Readers and individuals in general conversation in fact very commonly automatically employ context and related background knowledge to infer meaning (that is, fill in the blanks) that is not implicitly stated (Catts & Kamhi, 1999; Singer, 1990; Vargo, 2008).

Memory

If you ask someone if she has a good memory, that individual likely may reflect on how well she recalls details of events over a period of time, or how well she can memorize information to be recalled when needed. When asked about a child's memory abilities, a parent may describe in positive terms how his child often remembers details of past events or activities that he himself can barely remember, subsequently believing the child must have a good memory. Now, the ability to recall previously learned information or past events usually involves specific aspects of memory functions such as long-term memory retrieval and episodic or semantic memory processes (Baddeley, 2013; Gazzaniga, 2000; Kahana, 2012; Squire & Zola, 2000). Those cognitive functions, however, are only several aspects of the many components of memory processes and abilities (Ashcraft, 1989; Baddeley, 2013; Kandel et al., 2000; Kahana, 2012; Kolb & Wishaw, 2009; Wickelgren, 1981).

As discussed in Chapter 1, human beings at the cognitive and various physiological levels can be understood as information-processing organisms that interactively utilize the brain, the central nervous system, and related physical senses (Kalat, 2004; Kandel et al., 2000; Kolb & Wishaw, 2009; Shaffer & Kipp, 2009). Those information-processing capacities also interactively utilize components of memory systems and functions in virtually all processes of human cognition and learning (Ashcraft, 1989; Baddeley, 2013; Goswami, 2008; Kandel et al., 2000; Kahana, 2012; Kolb & Wishaw, 2009).

Many components of memory processes and functions can all be considered as aspects of human information processing. Some of those functions include sensory memory, short-term memory, working memory, long-term memory, and declarative memories. Each type of memory has its own particular mode of operation. The interactive actions of the various memory functions contribute to all learning and memory processes, including the establishment of long-term memories (Baddeley, 2013; Kahana, 2012; Lieberman, 2011).

Developmental delays in memory functions can dramatically affect learning and performance of many academic skills sets, including reading abilities, written language capabilities, and applied math skills and knowledge (Brady, Shankweiler, & Mann, 1983; Feifer & DeFina, 2000; Kibby, 2009; Miller, 2011; Mrazik, Bender, & Makovichuk, 2010; Sousa, 2008; Torgeson, 1988; Torgeson & Houck, 1990; Torgeson, Wagner, Rashotte, & Hecht, 1997; Vargo, 2007; Vargo, Grosser, & Spafford, 1995; Vargo, Young, & Vargo, 2004; Vargo et al., 2008; Vargo, Judah, & Young, 2010; Wolf, 1991). Memory functions can also change across the life span and can be altered as a result of neurophysiological trauma (Arnstein & Brown, 2005; Kandel et al., 2000; Lezak et al., 2004; Rypma & D'Esposito, 2000).

Sensory Memory

Every elementary schoolchild learns that we have five primary senses, which include sight, hearing, smell, taste, and touch (Carter, 2009; Kalat, 2004; Moore & Dalley, 1999). It is notable that each of the sensory processes involves a memory component known as sensory memory (Baddeley, 2013; Kahana, 2012; Kandel et al., 2000). Sensory memory is the shortest-term element of memory, and it has the ability to retain impressions of sensory information after the original stimuli have ended (Baddeley, 2013). For example, when you look at an object, the physical apparatus of your visual system initially receives and physically processes the information through a cascade of physiological processes, transforming environmental light waves into internal bioelectrical information (Kalat, 2004; Moore & Dalley, 1999). You then very briefly process and remember that information as a sensory memory. That sensory memory is, however, extremely brief, lasting approximately between one-fifth and half a second after the initial physiological visual perception (Baddeley, 2013; Kandel et al., 2000). This process happens automatically and with no conscious effort or control on your part. Further, you cannot rehearse the short-term memory (e.g., keep repeating it) to hold the sensory memory longer. Indeed, a sensory memory is an ultra-short-term cognitive event that ends (or decays) very quickly (Baddeley, 2013; Gazzaniga, 2000). The sensory memory for visual stimuli (sight) is also known as the iconic memory; the memory for aural stimuli (hearing) is also known as the echoic memory; and sensory memory for touch as also known as haptic memory.

What, then, is the importance of such a brief cognitive event as a sensory memory? Well, we can consider the sensory memory as a kind of buffer between actual physical sensory stimuli and concurrent memory functions. The sensory memory lasts for such a brief period of time that it is often understood as more of a perceptual process. Nevertheless, sensory memory is a component of memory that is an essential step for the subsequent storing of information in short-term memory (Ashcraft, 1989; Baddeley, 2013; Gazzaniga, 2000).

Through evolutionary processes, human brains are designed to process only information that is perceived to be of later use or value (Lieberman, 2011). Sensory memory information is either cognitively selected to be processed to another level (e.g., into short-term memory), or the information immediately decays and is completely forgotten (Baddeley, 2000; Rumelhart & Norman, 1983). So how does the brain select which sensory memory information is retained through further memory functions? Interestingly, the neurodevelopmental construct of attention plays an important role in that process. By utilizing active and conscious attentional processes, the brain can then effectively filter in or out information very briefly stored in sensory memory. As such, as in the various proposed models of human intelligence, attentional processes are an important component of virtually all stages of learning and memory activities and functions, especially in the process of the selection and transference of sensory memories (Ashcraft, 1989; Baddeley, 2013; Gazzaniga, 2000; Kandel et al., 2000).

Short-Term Memory and Working Memory

Consider the last time you needed to obtain a number to make a phone call. You may have used an actual phone book, searched it online, or used a phone-based search option. In any case, after obtaining the number, unless you immediately wrote the number down, you almost certainly needed to remember it for at least a few seconds until you could actually place the call. To do so, you most likely facilitated temporarily remembering the number by repeating it to yourself (also referred to as rehearsing the information), which held the number in your consciousness until you were able to dial it. Seconds after dialing the number and beginning the next step in your communication process, the number likely was extinguished from your memory. Actually, you never really learned the number in that scenario. What you did was briefly hold the number in your short-term memory.

As you are reading this sentence, you are using short-term memory processes to hold on to the initial information in the sentence while you continue reading the rest of the sentence (Ashcraft, 1989; Baddeley, 2013). When you are performing a mathematical calculation task that involves carrying over numbers across calculation columns, you will do so partially by utilizing integrative cognitive functions that include short-term memory (Matlin, 1989; Sousa, 2008). When you and another individual are having a conversation and sharing an effective communication experience, short-term memory capacities are helping to facilitate that process (Matlin, 1989).

Short-term memory can be understood as a cognitive memory function that allows us to both remember and process information simultaneously (Ashcraft, 1989; Kellogg, 2007). Those processes, however, occur within a short period of time, typically 10–15 seconds. In addition, short-term memory functions have been demonstrated to hold relatively small amounts of information, typically seven items or less (Cohen, Eysenck, & LeVoi, 1986; Matlin, 1989).

Information held in short-term memory quickly disappears completely unless an individual makes a conscious effort to move the information to long-term memory storage, or if other situations and related processes occur. For instance, repetition of information over time, such as dialing a specific telephone number over a period of days or weeks, may eventually facilitate the transformation of that information into a long-term memory, which an individual then may experience as a remembered item (Ashcraft, 1986; Cohen et al., 1986; Matlin, 1989). The process of transferring information from short-term to long-term memory storage may involve other interactive cognitive functions, such as associating certain information with other information, as in the utilization of mnemonic strategies for memorization. Another effective process for learning and memorizing involves the use of meaning and context to encode (store) specific units of information, such as when historical data (e.g., historical, names, dates, battles) are more successfully initially learned and then available for recall when they are processed in the context of a written (story) or visual (movie) narrative.

Working memory is another aspect of short-term memory, and the terms are often used interchangeably. The models of working memory include interactive cognitive components such as attention, executive functions, and various memory looping processes that allow for the concurrent holding, processing, and manipulation of information in short-term memory storage (Baddeley, 2013; Kahana, 2012). Consider the common student task of taking notes or dictation. While a teacher is verbally presenting information, perhaps using concurrent multiple modalities such as speaking and visual aids, a student in a dictation process needs to initially attend to the information and then hold it in short-term memory. The student has a very brief amount of time to write down what he or she is hearing, most often in a shorthand format summarizing what was said. While those two concurrent processes are occurring, the student must also listen to new information constantly being presented. In addition, the student must instantaneously decide which points being presented are most salient and need to be written down. In other words, the apparently simple task of taking lecture notes is actually a very complex process of interactive memory (and visual-motor) functions.

Long-Term Memory

Consider again parents who may describe their child as having a good memory because the child often remembers details of past events or activities that they themselves can barely remember. Those parents are referring to their child's long-term memory, which, in this case, is the ability to recall various types of information regarding details of past experiences and events.

Long-term memory involves the storage and retrieval of information over a long period of time (Baddeley, 2013; Lezak et al., 2004). While sensory memory and short-term memory functions are temporary processes, long-term memory can be considered as the permanent storage of information. The processes, then, of long-term memory functions also include the various ways of retrieving information in long-term memory stores (Baddeley, 2013; Lezak et al., 2004). What we all typically perceive as remembering (whether it be recalling events, rote facts, or many other types of information) actually involves a complex process of information processing, encoding (storing), and retrieval.

Memories temporarily held in short-term memory can become long-term memory through the process known as consolidation, which most typically involves the rehearsal (repetition) of short-term memory data, as well as the establishment of meaningful associations of information initially held in short-term memory to also facilitate effective transfer of information to long-term memory stores (Ashcraft, 1989; Baddeley, 2013; Lezak et al., 2004; Levine 2002; Lieberman, 2011; Kahana, 2012; Kandel et al., 2000).

To enhance the conceptualization of the complex processes of information storage and retrieval (learning and memory), the analogy of filing information in file cabinets may be helpful. Consider the office of a very active business (perhaps a dentist or doctor's office) that needs to have information stored and readily available when needed. Such an office today likely involves a combination of both physical paper files and computer-based files. To have information readily accessible in either format, a structured system typically involving organizing and storing information in alphabetical order may be utilized. More specifically, the process may involve initially choosing (attending to) what information is to be filed at a given moment, deciding how to organize the information (likely alphabetically), and then doing so (analogous to processing cognitive information), perhaps walking a short distance into another room to the actual physical file cabinet while briefly continuing to remember the task at hand (analogous to short-term memory), physically storing the information in the actual file cabinet (analogous to transferring short-term memory storage to long-term memory storage through a process of cognitive encoding), and retrieving the information when needed from the file cabinet (analogous to retrieving information from long-term memory storage). What happens, however, if the information is not stored in a well-organized and categorical manner? For instance, on a busy day some files may be just tossed into the cabinet arbitrarily to be later organized alphabetically. Those files would likely be less accessible if needed in a hurry, and a more random search process of reaching in for the files would likely be ineffective. In other words, ineffective organizing, processing, and initial storing of information results in stored information that is less easily retrievable and accessible.

Types of Long-Term Memory

Long-term memory-based information can be categorized in various ways, based on the nature and functions of a memory (Ashcraft, 1989; Groth-Marnat, 2000; Levine, 2002; Lieberman, 2011). For instance, information in long-term memory can be further described as explicit or implicit memory. Explicit memories are conscious memories such as events in our lives, subjective experiences, and information that has been deliberately studied. Implicit memories are unconscious memory functions generally encompassing a range of associated and integrated cognitive and physiological learned tasks such as driving a car or typing on a keyboard.

Explicit long-term memories, based on most current models of memory processes in the neurosciences, can be further categorized as declarative memories, which can be further divided into even more specific categories of episodic and semantic memories. While declarative memory patterns can be understood as general facts and events in one's life, episodic memories specifically refer to representations of our memory and recollections of autobiographic experiences and specific events in time that we serially reconstruct not only cognitively, but with associated emotions and contexts. In contrast, semantic memories are permanently stored components of acquired general factual knowledge such as learned facts and concepts, as well as contextual experiences associated with such information (Figure 2.1; Ashcraft, 1989; Baddeley, 2013; Lezak et al., 2004; Lieberman, 2011; Kahana, 2012; Kandel et al., 2000).

FIGURE 2.1. HUMAN MEMORY FUNCTIONS

Sensory Memory (*<1 second*)	Short-Term/ Working Memory (*<1 minute*)	Long-Term Memory (*Permanent Memory*)

	Explicit Memory (*Conscious*)	Implicit Memory (*Unconscious*)

	Declarative Memory (*Events and Facts*)	Procedural Memory (*Learned Motor Skill Sets*)

	Episodic Memory (*Experiences and Events*)	Semantic Memory (*Facts and Concepts*)

Schematic Memory

The fields of cognitive psychology, developmental psychology, and the neurosciences have contributed other models of cognition and learning relative to long-term memory theories, known as schematic memory processes and schema theory. Schemas can be understood as packets of information stored in long-term memory that are derived from past experiences and learning, and include memories of general knowledge, situations, and events (Cohen et al., 1986). The concept of schemas was first posited in the early 1930s (Bartlett, 1932), and those earlier cognitive models of learning provided a theoretical foundation for evolving theories of schematic functions in memory processes, as well as for the pivotal developmental theories of Jean Piaget (1972; Rumelhart & Norman, 1983).

Schematic-based models of learning and related theories of memory emphasize that prior stored knowledge in the form of schematic memory representations has an effect on the understanding, acquisition, and encoding of new information (Cohen et al., 1986; Levine, 2002; Piaget, 1972; Rayner & Pollatsek, 1989; Rumelhart & Norman, 1983). Simply put, the more knowledge an individual already possesses (factual and conceptual) about a given topic, the easier and more efficient it likely is for that individual to understand and assimilate new information about that specific content area. Conversely, an individual who is attempting to learn and memorize information (both factually and conceptually) about a topic that he or she has little or no prior information on may find it more difficult to initially process and understand the new information, since there is no foundation of previous related information that could provide a contextual framework for new information acquisition and learning to occur (Ashcraft, 1989; Levine, 2002; Matlin, 1989).

Temporal-Sequential Ordering

The general neurodevelopmental construct of temporal-sequential ordering involves the perception, understanding, and application of time and sequences. The integration of such cognitive functions and processes provide a foundation for many educational abilities and academic tasks (Berninger & Richards, 2002; Levine, 2002; Spafford & Grosser, 1996). For instance, when young children learn to recite and memorize the alphabet, they are utilizing temporal-sequential ordering abilities (Fawcett & Nicolson, 2001; Levine, 1995). Mathematical functions and processes across all grade levels may also involve complex interactions of temporal-sequential cognitive abilities (Barnes et al., 2010; Berninger & Richards, 2002; Maricle et al., 2010; Montague & Jitendra, 2006; Sousa, 2008).

Consider that generating a writing project, especially in the higher academic grades, involves considerable sequential ordering and organization skills and capabilities (Feifer & DeFina, 2002). How does one initially organize proposed main topics for a narrative theme? How does a writer organize and logically sequence developing and supportive factual and thematic information? How does an author of a writing project research, organize, and sequentially outline information obtained from multiple resources? When considering these factors, one can appreciate the extensive and complex integrated temporal-sequential ordering processes that are necessary components of most writing tasks (Jongmans, 2005; Feifer & DeFina, 2002).

From remembering telephone numbers and addresses to being able to tell time on a clock, to learning an educational song, to solving multistep high school equations and word problems, to being able to track and understand the plot of a story, the neurodevelopmental construct of temporal-sequential ordering is an important contributing component of learning and understanding (Barnes et al., 2010; Berninger & Richards, 2002; Fawcett & Nicolson, 2001; Jongmans, 2005; Levine, 1995; Montague & Jitendra, 2006; Sousa, 2008).

Spatial Ordering

The general developmental construct of spatial ordering involves the ability to perceive, organize, and apply visual-spatial information. Developmental deficits that involve spatial ordering functions and processes can manifest as difficulties in orienting to objects in space, and difficulties with directions (Kurtz, 2007; Levine, 2002).

Developmental delays that involve spatial ordering processes can manifest in a range of difficulties involving relatively basic to quite complex tasks and processes. For instance, fundamental academic skills, critical for early writing and math development, commonly involve concepts such as "left" and "right" and using margins and rows when organizing and understanding written and mathematical information. More complex tasks involving integrated spatial ordering processes could range from completing simple puzzles to assembling complicated mechanical devices. Effective general time management, recognizing faces, visually discriminating between different coins, visualizing the possible location of lost objects, and assimilating the general thematic meaning of a long fact-based story all also include components of spatial ordering constructs and related integrated cognitive functions and processes (Chittooran & Tait, 2005; Crawford, 2007; Emerson & Babtie, 2010; Feifer & DeFina, 2002; Henderson, 2012; Jones, 2005; Kurtz, 2007; Yeo, 2005).

Developmental delays and deficits in various areas of spatial ordering and processing can also be common in individuals with nonverbal learning disability. This syndrome involves problems with general visual-spatial processing and awareness, and related neurocognitive deficits involving temporal-sequential ordering and spatial ordering (Palombo, 2006; Rourke, 1995b). Nonverbal learning disability also commonly includes difficulties and deficits in other integrated nurodevelopmental constructs, such as psychomotor coordination, language (semantic language, sarcasm, and understanding of higher-order language concepts), tactile (touch) and visual attention and perception, and social functioning (e.g., reading others' facial cues, mannerisms, prosodic information, or body language context) (Palombo, 2006; Rourke, 1989, 1995b).

Neuromotor Functions

Neuromotor functions include all integrated and interrelated fine motor, gross motor, and visual-motor skills, which are important across a wide range of learning and educational processes (Ball, 2002; Boon, 2010; Chambers, Sugden, & Sinani, 2005; Drew & Creek, 2005; Wade, Johnson, & Mally, 2005; Meece & Daniels, 2008).

Developmental theories and related psychological models have provided a foundation of theories and stages of human developmental functions and processes across the life span (Gallahue, 1992; Jones, 2005; Kurtz, 2007; Piaget, 1972; Pressley & McCormick, 2007; Sugden & Chambers, 2005). Such theories and models include integrated stages of cognitive, motor, and social developmental processes (Goswami, 2008; Spreen, Risser, & Edgell, 1995; Sprinthall & Sprinthall, 1990). Foundational theories posited by Jean Piaget outline early stages of such integrated developmental processes (Piaget, 1972; Sprinthall & Sprinthall, 1990). Developing neuromotor functions, according to Piaget's theories, are primary during the first 2 years of life. Piaget posited that during that period of a child's life and development, which he named the sensorimotor stage, an infant's knowledge of the world is primarily limited to his or her sensory perceptions and motor activities, and developing understanding and learning are strongly related to simple motor responses caused by sensory stimuli that a child utilizes to gain understanding of the environment and the self.

While neuromotor processes (including developing fine motor and gross motor skills) appear to play a primary role in early childhood development and learning, they continue to be important components of learning and understanding across later developmental stages and indeed across the human life span (Drew & Creek, 2005; Shah & Donald, 1986; Walsh et al., 2013). While a child may be utilizing integrated visual-spatial and spatial-ordering cognitive constructs while engaged in a puzzle-solving task, such a pursuit also typically involves an important degree of neuromotor functions that cooperatively integrate with other various cognitive and motor functions (Ball, 2002; Jones, 2005; Jongmans, 2005; Kirby & Drew, 2003).

Consider that many tasks, from producing written language (by hand or computer keyboard) to playing a musical instrument, to performing virtually any athletic activity involves a complex integration of neuromotor functions and cognitive processes that also facilitate visual-spatial and spatial ordering constructs, and in some cases (such as the production of written language) also incorporate higher-order thinking and reasoning capabilities (Jones, 2005; Ripley, 2001; Wade et al., 2005).

Levine (2002) has presented a model of human motor functions that includes five distinctly related neurodevelopmental subconstructs, including gross motor functions, fine motor functions, graphomotor functions (writing), oromotor functions (speaking), and musical motor functions. Levine identifies gross motor functions as involving integrated activities of larger muscles, such as in an athletic activity. In contrast, fine motor functions (also often referred to as eye-hand coordination) more typically involve tasks requiring manual dexterity such as threading a needle or clipping fingernails. While fine motor abilities are arguably important components of the physical act of forming letters, the general academic tasks of writing and written language development encompass more complex integrated neuromotor functions that fall under Levine's subconstruct of graphomotor skills (Mody & Silliman, 2008a; Sousa, 2008; Zemelman, Daniels, & Hyde, 2005). For instance, some students with graphomotor deficits may write inefficiently and poorly because their fingers do not coordinate well with the flow of thoughts and language. Such neurodevelopmentally delayed students may also have gaps and deficits in motor visualization or motor sequential memory functions that are also important components of integrated writing skills.

Oromotor processes involve integrated facial muscular and speech production functions that facilitate a range of oral communication abilities, including speaking and aspects of oral language production (Shah & Donald, 1986). When a student participates in a class discussion, oromotor functions come strongly into play. When a young learner attempts to sound out phonological and phonemic information, oromotor processes are strongly involved. When a baby or a toddler is learning to repeat verbal sounds and subsequently learn and assimilate language, oromotor functions are critical to the process (Freeman & Soltanifar, 2010; Geuze, 2005; Walsh et al., 2013).

Musical motor output can involve a wide range of integrated neuromotor functions that include various oromotor, fine motor, and in some cases gross motor functions (Gueze, 2005). Different musical activities can range from singing to playing the piano, the trombone, and the drums. Such diverse musical expressions involve differing complex sequences of neuromotor abilities depending on the physical and cognitive skills and functions required.

FIGURE 2.2. THE HUMAN MOTOR FUNCTION SYSTEM

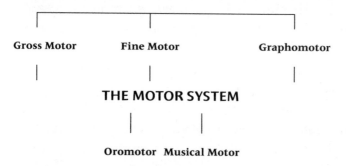

Social Cognition

If asked, many individuals may describe social skills as being important in many aspects of life. It would likely be hard to find many individuals who believe that at least a reasonable amount of interpersonal abilities are not important in the process of navigating through the world socially and at times vocationally. But how important are social and interpersonal abilities in learning and effective functioning across multiple educational environments? How important are social skills in learning in many life activities that are not directly focused on relationship development?

Consider that what many individuals understand and perceive as social and interpersonal talents can in a neurodevelopmental construct model be more comprehensively understood as social intelligence. As such, from learning and neurodevelopmental perspectives, individual strengths in aspects of social and interpersonal functioning can be framed as components of cognition, intelligence, and as a specific neurodevelopmental construct (Gardner, 1983; Levine, 2002).

Levine (2002) posited that an often underestimated and even overlooked component of learning is the ability to succeed in social relationships with peers, parents, and teachers. While some learners may be strong in other neurodevelopmental functions, inabilities to effectively develop positive peer relationships, work in groups, or cope effectively with peer pressure and other social system functions can significantly interfere with an individual's ability to effectively learn as well as function across various educational and vocational environments (Crawford, 2007; Vargo, 2008).

Difficulties with social cognition and applied social intelligence often are components of other profiles of neurodevelopmental disorders and learning disabilities. For instance, individuals with cognitive impairments in visual-spatial processing (commonly seen in nonverbal learning disabilities), higher-order language functions, or temporal sequencing dysfunctions (or a combination of those neurodevelopmental deficits) may frequently have difficulties with interpersonal communications and functioning partially as the result of ineffective and impaired cognitive processing capacities (Gualtieri, Koriath, Bourgondien, & Saleeby, 1983; Cohen, Davine, &

Meloche-Kelly, 1989; Kuder, 2003; Love & Thompson, 1988; Palombo, 2006; Rourke & Fuerts, 1991).

Consider the deceptively simple act of two individuals having a conversation. When you are face to face with another individual and you are both engaged in an interactive verbal dialogue, the communication and information processes are likely occurring at many different levels and across multiple interactive cognitive functions (Vargo, 2008). To partially understand what your speaking partner is saying, you must process spoken language at the word, semantic, and syntactic levels, and at higher levels of language involving inferential processing and contextual understanding (Catts & Kamhi, 1999). Ongoing communications are also, however, occurring at various nonverbal levels. Nuances of meaning and understanding are being expressed through facial expressions, varying voice pitches and tone (called verbal prosody), hand and body gestures, and even more subtle interpersonal signs, perhaps at times below levels of conscious awareness. While both communicants are continuously processing and understanding multiple levels of verbal and nonverbal communication, each is also processing individual information at sensory and physiological levels. Many of those processing functions are happening below awareness thresholds (Borod, 2000; Lane & Nadel, 2000; Suchy, 2011). In fact, so much information is continuously being processed at so many different levels that much of that data needs to be perceptually screened and prioritized, or we would all likely be constantly overwhelmed with sensory and physiological processes (Ashcraft, 1989; Cozolino, 2006). When considering the breadth, levels, and complexity of functions that occur in even the most basic of communication exchanges, it is not difficult to understand how developmental disabilities that interfere with any involved processing capacities can adversely affect perceptions, understanding, and communications at varying levels and degrees. As an example of how interrelated cognitive and processing functions can impair an individual's social and interpersonal capacities, consider the following case example.

CASE STUDY 2.1: JERRY

Jerry is a 13-year-old student with an assessed overall average range of intellectual functioning, but with specific neurodevelopmental deficits in higher-order language processing and understanding, as well as cognitive processing deficits in visual-spatial processing and organization. In addition to his recognized learning and academic difficulties based on his individual profile of cognitive functioning and learning styles, Jerry's teachers and parents are very concerned about his ability to function socially and interpersonally. His current classroom teacher has repeatedly observed that when Jerry is talking with peers, he often is unaware of and subsequently violates norms of personal space between individuals, and his peers frequently react to him negatively. When Jerry's classmates respond to him with notably and visibly irritated and even angry visual expressions, it has been repeatedly observed that Jerry often does not accurately visually process and integrate the communicative information that others are providing through facial expressions and body gestures and language. Jerry misreads and misunderstands the communications and responses of others and continues to respond and behave accordingly.

His teacher and parents also have observed that Jerry often misperceives combined and often subtle visual and language interactions and communications from his peers. For instance, he often misses it when others make sarcastic comments. When that happens, he may fail to process and integrate telltale visual cues such as eye rolling and smirking. He may misunderstand prosodic information (e.g., tone of voice) and subsequently misinterpret a sarcastic comment such as "nice hat" as an actual compliment. His teachers and his parents have learned through observation that when explaining information and giving him directions, Jerry must be provided with nonambiguous language and words as much as possible to best facilitate his accurate understanding. For instance, if he is told to "go outside and draw a bucket of water from the garden hose for the flowers out back," Jerry may become quite confused by such a directive single sentence that is potentially semantically, syntactically, and inferentially confusing.

Jerry's parents note that their son often has difficulties understanding the connections between multiple interrelated events and subsequent outcomes involving the responses and behaviors of other. He often seems to have difficulties integrating and synthesizing multiple points of information and events to understand cause and effect actions and reactions in others and in the environment.

Jerry has been seeing a therapist for individual counseling to help him to better understand his issues, social difficulties, and his related emotional responses. His counselor, while well clinically trained, has expressed to Jerry's parents that at times she does not fully understand the connections between his learning and processing disabilities and his capacity to adequately perceive and understand his world at a developmentally appropriate level.

Higher-Order Cognition and Functions

Can you consider, compare, and explain the conceptual differences between objects? How does a professional therapist approach an intervention process between emotionally conflicted individuals? How does one critically consider and assess if a written story is literal or a metaphor? What cognitive capabilities does a student utilize when integrating knowledge or grammar and punctuation rules while writing a paragraph? What mental functions are used in creative processes such as writing a poem or creating a musical composition? All of these situations require various aspects and components of higher-order cognition and functions.

Learning and thinking processes that involve creative and critical thinking, analogical reasoning, and concept formation can decrease an overreliance on rote memory across many academic tasks, and may generally positively enhance educational experiences for competent learners (Sousa, 2001; Zemelman et al., 2005).

The developmental constructs of higher-order cognition and functions include the ability to understand and implement steps involved in problem solving, understanding and applying new areas and strategies in learning, and thinking creatively (Mody & Silliman, 2008a). More specifically demonstrated higher-order functions that have been researched (Sousa, 2001; Zemelman et al., 2005) include the following:

- The ability to understand concepts, including applied mathematical concepts and language concepts
- The ability to problem solve across various tasks, including visual-spatial processes and language and nonverbal patterns
- The ability to develop divergent and creative thinking models

In convergent thought processes, a learner may obtain information from multiple sources (such as researching information about a topic on the Internet) and then strive to integrate that information to problem solve or consolidate a new concept. In a more divergent thinking scenario, an individual is likely to focus more on considering and understanding multiple possibilities of a concept or problem.

- The ability to think in analogies. For instance, a learner may need such a mental skill set to understand metaphorical stories that provide examples and teachings.
- The ability to conceptualize classifications. Consider that oranges and apples are things that can be eaten, and that

they also both fall into the category of fruits. The latter association requires a somewhat higher level of understanding in terms of a specific classification (fruit), as well as a greater ability to conceptualize complex and abstract concepts that connect both of those objects.

• The ability to integrate information. Learned information has minimal value if an individual cannot effectively organize it, assimilate it, and demonstrate knowledge of it. In other words, how does an individual take many components of information and concepts and put them all together?

To begin with, higher-order thinking involves the ability to think and reason in complex patterns. Higher-order neurodevelopmental functions involve an individual's ability to overall functionally integrate and assimilate many brain systems to achieve degrees of concept formation (Goswami, 2008). In addition, higher-order thinking and integrated cognitive functions strongly involve various aspects of mental abilities known as executive functions (Yeager & Yeager, 2013).

The executive functions involve a range of cognitive skills and capabilities that allow one to coordinate and integrate more fundamental knowledge and skills in order to pursue particular goals. The executive functions are not primarily concerned with what one actually knows and can do. They are primarily related to how and whether one is able to use knowledge and skills in goal-directed ways. The executive functions include such crucial multifaceted learning skill sets such as goal formulation and planning, the generation and organization of learning strategies, attentional control, the generation and flexible shifting of mental sets, the inhibition of impulsive responses, and the regulation and monitoring of one's own performance (Dawson & Guare, 2004; Barkley, 1997; Goldberg, 2001; Vargo et al., 2010; Yeager & Yeager, 2013).

Chapter 3

INTELLECTUAL DEVELOPMENTAL DISORDER

How smart are you? That simple question may be deceptively difficult to answer, as many individuals may reactively ask how one is defining the concept "smart." For instance, are you good at understanding and solving various types of problems? Are you good at understanding and even memorizing what you may read? Are you good with your hands and good at fixing things? Do you enjoy using calculus and solving differential equations? Are you an accomplished musician? How comfortable and effective are you at interacting with people and navigating social situations? Are you athletically inclined? Many models and theories of intelligence posit that most of these abilities and skill sets, some of them more typically referred to as talents, are actually various facets and types of intelligence (Cattell, 1943; Gardner, 1983; Ginsburg & Opper, 1987; Gruber & Voneche, 1995; Meece & Daniels, 2008; Piaget, 1972; Pressley & McCormick, 2007; Sattler, 2001; Sprinthall & Sprinthall, 1990; Sternberg & Berg, 1986; Terman, 1921; Wechsler, 1958, 2001, 2002).

To provide a frame of reference for understanding intellectual disability, the notion of intelligence may be understood as the general mental capability of an individual. General intelligence involves but is not limited to the ability to reason, plan, solve problems, think abstractly, comprehend complex ideas, learn quickly, and learn from experience (Armstrong, Hangauer, & Nadeau, 2012; Mervis & John, 2010; Pennington, 2009; Rondal et al., 2004; Sattler, 2001; Sprinthall & Sprinthall, 1990; Yeates et al., 2010). Intelligence as a quantitative measure is generally understood to be represented by intelligence quotient (IQ) scores obtained from specific standardized tests given by trained professionals. Intellectual disability is generally thought to be present if an individual has an IQ test score of approximately 70 or below (Armstrong et al., 2012; Drozdick, Wahlstrom, Zhu, & Weiss, 2012; Flanagan & Harrison, 2012; Sattler, 2001; Schalock, 2009; Sprinthall & Sprinthall, 1990).

INTELLECTUAL DISABILITY

Intellectual disability, also known as intellectual developmental disorder, is a neurodevelopmental disability that by definition occurs before age 18 and is also characterized by significant limitations in intellectual functioning and adaptive behavior as expressed in conceptual, social, and practical adaptive skills (AAIDD, 2014; American Psychiatric Association, 2013; Schalock, 2009). Intellectual developmental disorder is diagnosed through the use of standardized tests of intelligence and adaptive behavior.

The definition of intellectual disability used most often in the United States comes from the American Association on Intellectual and Developmental Disabilities (AAIDD, 2014; Schalock, 2009). The American Psychiatric Association (2013), in the *DSM-5*, currently establishes a diagnosis of intellectual developmental disorder under the more general diagnostic category of neurodevelopmental disorders. The World Health Organization (2014) recognizes intellectual disabilities under the general category of mental retardation, with varying degrees of the disability. The three diagnostic models currently posited by AAIDD, the American Psychiatric Association (APA), and the World Health Organization are generally consistent and in concert with the AAIDD definition that is used in the United States.

Intellectual disabilities can be understood as developmental deficits in general mental abilities—more specifically, in cognitive areas involving reasoning, abstract thinking, judgment, problem solving, academic functioning, and even one's ability to learn and grow intellectually through experience (Mervis & John, 2010; Pennington, 2009; Rondal et al., 2004; Yeates et al., 2010). An important component of an intellectual disabilities diagnosis is an impairment in general adaptive functioning, such as a developmentally appropriate ability to manage self-care and self-safety habits (Batshaw, 1997; American Psychiatric Association, 2013). For older individuals with clinical profiles of primary intellectual deficiencies, deficits in adaptive functioning typically also include significant difficulties in areas involving social and interpersonal functioning, occupational functioning, and independence in living and related life skills (Hassiotis et al., 2010; Whitaker, 2013). Causes of intellectual developmental disorder span a range of genetic and medical etiologies (Mervis & John, 2010; Rondal et al., 2004; Yeates et al., 2010).

DIAGNOSING INTELLECTUAL DISABILITIES

The growth and abilities of children typically follow general patterns and age-related stages. As children mature into the preschool and early elementary years, many cognitive and motor functions emerge and develop along a continuum of progressive abilities. Those patterns, however, can naturally vary between individuals within typical functional ranges, and it is important to understand that some variability can be expected in many areas of child development. For instance, children by 12 months typically begin to imitate different speech sounds and develop several words such as "mama" and "dada," but the ability to produce speech at that age may vary between individual children and siblings (Gleason, 1989; Kuder, 2003; Meece & Daniels, 2008; Pressley & McCormick, 2007).

The integration of those many aspects of child development as children physically mature allow for a natural progression of a child's ability to function appropriately for his or her age across environments, such as at home or in early educational placements. For example, early language abilities progress through more complex stages of language understanding and usage. Various fine-motor and gross-motor functions progressively develop. General thinking, reasoning, and understanding abilities increase with physical maturity (Kuder, 2003; Mastergeorge, 2013; Meece & Daniels, 2008; Pressley & McCormick, 2007; Sprinthall & Sprinthall, 1990). A knowledge and understanding of general developmental considerations and milestones are important to parents and medical and education professionals involved with young children, and can also be important when concern is raised that a child may be developing in atypical ways.

IF INTELLECTUAL DISABILITY IS SUSPECTED

A parent, physician, or early child educator may initially become concerned about the possibility of a child having an intellectual disability. Perhaps a toddler's speech and communication skills development seems atypical, or the general daily functioning and social abilities of a preschool-age child do not appear to be age appropriate. While such developmental delays may not be related to an actual intellectual disability, in such a case it is appropriate to follow up with appropriate professionals.

Since an intellectual disability in a child is defined by two major symptoms (significant limitations in intellectual functioning and related mental abilities concurrent with developmental delays in general functioning in social abilities and practical life skills), the diagnostic process typically includes multiple steps and professionals from various disciplines. A thorough assessment to diagnose a possible intellectual disability in a child needs to include the following components:

- A comprehensive medical exam
- A social and familial history
- interviews with primary caregivers and preschool educators
- An educational history (if child is older)
- Psychological testing to assess intellectual functioning
- Assessment of adaptive functioning across various areas and domains
- Social and behavioral observations of the child across environments
- Possible genetic and neurological testing

Of these various diagnostic components, the assessment of intellectual functioning and adaptive functioning are of primary importance, as deficits in these two global areas of functioning are defining features of an intellectual disability (AAIDD, 2014; APA, 2013; Hodapp & Dykens, 2004, 2012; Mervis & John, 2010; Rondal et al., 2004). As such, a more comprehensive understanding of cognitive and adaptive functioning is valuable to all individuals raising such concerns for a child.

DEGREES OF INTELLECTUAL DISABILITY

An intellectual disability, like many other disorders, is not an all-or-nothing condition, but occurs along a continuum, with varying degrees of functioning across cognitive, social, and adaptive abilities. In fact, the American Association on Intellectual and Developmental Disabilities (2014) and the American

Psychiatric Association use specific severity codes to better clarify how an individual with an intellectual disability functions along a range of mental and adaptive capabilities. The *Diagnostic and Statistical Manual of Mental Disorders*, Fifth Edition (*DSM-5*) includes the categories of mild, moderate, severe, and profound intellectual disability (APA, 2013). Diagnostic decisions regarding the severity of a disability are typically based on conceptual, social, and practical life domains and functioning.

Based on the current *DSM-5* classifications, individuals diagnosed with an intellectual disability within a mild range (which encompasses about 85% of individuals with the disability) will require educational and related areas of support across their lives. Children with mild disability are usually able to have their educational needs met in general public school settings with varying and individualized levels of academic and remedial interventions and accommodations and educational mainstreaming with typically developing students determined as best appropriate for each child (Hazlett et al., 2011; Hodapp & Dykens, 2004, 2012; Mervis & John, 2010). Adults with mild intellectual disability typically are mostly self-sufficient in adulthood if provided with minimal support services such as help with personal finances, transportation, and work life. In sum, many individuals with a diagnosed mild range of intellectual disability live independently within their communities with a minimal level of additional consistent support.

Individuals diagnosed with moderate intellectual disability (about 10% of individuals with the disability) in general will require higher degrees of supports and programming across their lives. Children with moderate disability are also usually able to have their educational needs met in general public school settings with varying and individualized levels of academic and remedial interventions and accommodations (Hodapp & Dykens, 2004, 2012). In general, students in the moderate ranges will require more intensive educational interventions, which may involve less educational mainstreaming with typically developing learners. Adults with moderate-range intellectual disability typically will also require more extensive supports and services to help them function in all aspects of their lives (Hassiotis et al., 2010).

Individuals diagnosed with a severe intellectual disability (about 3% to 4% of individuals with the disability) in general will require very high and consistent degrees of support and programming across their lives (Hassiotis et al., 2010). Children and adults with severe global intellectual deficits typically have limited communication skills and require extensive support in daily self-care activities. Children in this range may still be provided with educational programming in public school settings, but their individualized academic programming may be implemented entirely within special education classes and programs separate from mainstream classes (Rondal et al., 2004). Even more intensive levels of educational and multifaceted clinical services and supports will be necessary for children and adults with intellectual disabilities that fall within a profound range. Those in this category typically have extreme deficits in communication and language functions, and usually require 24-hour support and care for virtually all of their daily and living functions (Hassiotis et al., 2010; Rondal et al., 2004).

CAUSES OF INTELLECTUAL DISABILITY DISORDER

When parents are told that their child has an intellectual disability or any other neurodevelopmental disorder and related learning problems, an initial question might involve the cause of the disability. It is often difficult, however, to recognize a clear and definitive underlying cause of an intellectual disability, as many possible factors and conditions can contribute to these disorders. An intellectual disability may be the outcome of a number of different causes, and the actual etiology may ultimately not be able to be recognized. Some of those causes are preventable, but others are clearly not preventable. The factors that can result in an individual having an intellectual disability can be understood within four general categories: (1) genetic conditions, (2) psychiatric conditions, (3) medical conditions, and (4) acquired brain damage (Hagerman, 2011; Hazlett, Hammer, Hooper, & Kamphaus, 2011; Hodapp & Dykens, 2004; Mervis & John, 2010; Rondal et al., 2004).

Within the context of these factors, most common causes that result in an intellectual disability are Down syndrome and fragile X syndrome (which are genetic disorders), autism spectrum disorder (a psychiatric diagnosis), and the medical condition of fetal alcohol syndrome (Corbett & Gunther, 2011; Hagerman, 2011; Hazlett et al., 2011; Mattson & Vaurio, 2010).

Extensive medical and clinical knowledge may be needed to understand the scope of factors that can cause or contribute to intellectual disability. A general overview, however, of the most common conditions contributing to intellectual disability disorder will likely be of great value for educators and parents involved with the disability.

INTELLECTUAL DISABILITIES INVOLVING GENETIC CONDITIONS

Down Syndrome

Down syndrome is the most common genetic origin of intellectual disabilities. Some degree of general intellectual and cognitive impairment is present in all individuals with the syndrome. It is a genetic disorder with a distinct cause and a wide range of cognitive, learning, behavioral, and medical complications. Down syndrome is caused by an extra chromosome, which occurs because of an error in cell division during prenatal growth. The disorder can be inherited, but the majority of cases are not inherited and result from accidents in chromosomal distribution during prenatal development (Bivina, Moghaddam, & Wardinsky, 2013; Cook & Leventhal, 1992; Hazlett et al., 2011; Teeter & Semrud-Clikeman, 2007). The prevalence rates of Down syndrome internationally are approximately 8 out of every 10,000 births (Cocchi et al., 1995).

Individuals with Down syndrome have a specific pattern of physiological characteristics and symptoms, which include physical brain abnormalities that directly result in varying degrees of global intellectual impairments (within mild to profound ranges of intellectual disability), facial features including eyes with an atypical upward slant and white spots on the iris of the eye, a notably short neck and flat face, and a protrusion of the tongue that may increase with age (Bivina et al., 2013; Pueschel, 1992). The condition is also associated with possible cardiovascular issues and other medical problems related to vision, hearing, and neuromuscular conditions (Teeter & Semrud-Clikeman, 2007; Cicchetti & Beeghly, 1990).

The more typical physical features of Down syndrome are usually recognizable at birth. Also, the general physical features and degrees of intellectual impairment vary between individuals, resulting in a heterogeneous group of individuals with the disorder, and some physical traits may be evident in other medical and genetic conditions (Pueschel, 1992). Thus, genetic testing of a child with features of Down syndrome is appropriate to clarify a diagnosis or to obtain information regarding a possible differential diagnosis. The definitive diagnosis of Down syndrome requires a blood test called a chromosomal karyotype, and takes about two weeks to complete (Bivina et al., 2013; Goldstein & Reynolds, 2011; Hazlett et al., 2011).

Fragile X Syndrome

Fragile X syndrome, a genetic disorder associated with mild to severe and profound ranges of intellectual disability disorder, is considered to be the most common cause of inherited intellectual disabilities (Papilia & Olds, 1992; Teeter & Semrud-Clikeman, 2007; Wolf-Schein, 1992). Fragile X is the most common genetic cause of intellectual disabilities in males, and a significant cause in females. The disorder appears in families of every ethnic group and income level (Hagerman, 2011; Leigh, Hagerman, & Hessl, 2013; National Human Genome Research Institute, 2014).

Fragile X syndrome results from a change, or mutation, in a single gene, which can be passed from one generation to the next. The syndrome occurs because the mutated gene cannot produce enough of a protein that is needed by the body's cells, especially cells in the brain, to develop normally (Hodapp & Dykens, 2012; National Human Genome Research Institute, 2014). People with fragile X syndrome also share certain medical problems and many common physical characteristics (Chaste et al., 2012; Cornish, Turk, & Hagelman, 2008; De Vries, Halley, Oostra, & Niermeijer, 1994; Tovi, Buterbaugh, Love, & Visootsak, 2013). Fragile X is also often associated with difficulties in emotion and behavior, such as recurring episodes of tantrums, anxiety, and poor attentional control (Hagerman, 2011; Hodapp & Dykens, 2012; Leigh et al., 2013). The following outlines the most typical features and behaviors associated with fragile X syndrome:

Physical Features

Long face (prominent forehead and chin)

Long ears

Prominent ears

Hand calluses

Flat feet

Single Palmer crease of the hand

Large head circumference in babies

Double-jointed thumbs

Developmental motor delays

Physical tremors

Developmentally poor coordination

Hyperextensible finger joints

Cardiac murmur and other cardiac problems

Behavioral Features

Poor eye contact

Hand flapping

Hand biting

Developmental language delays

Verbal and behavioral perseverations

Verbal and physical outbursts

Tantrum behaviors

Attention problems

Hyperactivity

Shyness and social anxiety

Hypersensitivity to multiple sensory stimuli

Hypersensitivity to crowds and loud noises

Rett Syndrome

Rett syndrome is a genetic neurodevelopmental disorder that occurs almost exclusively in females, which commonly results in severe and profound levels of intellectual disability. It is a major cause of intellectual disability disorder in females (Brown & McMillan, 2011). The condition is a rare disorder, occurring in approximately 1 in 15,000 female births worldwide (Brown & McMillan, 2011; Hagberg, 1995; Percy, 2002). Rett syndrome is characterized by normal early growth and development followed by a slowing of development, intellectual disability, slowed brain and head growth, loss of purposeful use of the hands and distinctive hand movements, general motor dysfunctions and related walking problems, and seizures (Boa, Downs, Wong, Williams, & Leonard, 2013; Brown, McMillan, & Herschthal, 2005; Hanks, 1990; National Institute of Neurological Disorders and Stroke, 2008b).

The diagnosis of Rett syndrome will involve, in addition to an initial primary care pediatrician, a pediatric neurologist, a clinical geneticist, or a developmental pediatrician, or a combination of those medical professionals. Clinical and medical experts will observe for signs and symptoms during the child's early growth and development, and conduct ongoing evaluations of the child's physical and neurological status. A genetic test for the mutation on a child's X chromosome is also a typical component of the diagnostic process (Armstrong, 2005; Brown et al., 2005; Hunter, 2007; International Rett Syndrome Foundation, 2008).

It is important for parents and early childhood professionals to understand that babies with Rett syndrome appear to grow and behave normally for about the first 6 months of life. Children with the disorder typically begin to present specific signs and symptoms between 18 and 23 months of age. These signs and indications are as follows (Armstrong, 2005; Brown et al., 2005; Hagburg, 1995; Halbach et al., 2013; International Rett Syndrome Foundation, 2008; Percy, 2002; Mayo Clinic, 2014; Naidu, 1997; National Institute of Neurological Disorders and Stroke, 2008b; Van Acker, 1991):

- A slowing of physical growth and resulting notable delays in physical development. After an initial 6-month period of apparent normal development after birth, a child with Rett syndrome may exhibit a smaller than developmentally typical head size, concurrent with diminished levels of brain growth and development, which is often the first outward indication of the syndrome. As these children become older, delayed growth in other parts of the body becomes more evident.
- There is a notable diminishing of normal movement and coordination. The most significant loss of movement skills and general motor skills in a child with Rett syndrome usually begins to become apparent between 12 and 18 months of age. For instance, a parent may observe a decreased abil-

ity to crawl and walk, or may notice that a child has less control of hand movements such as grasping and holding than previously attained.

- Unusual eye movements. A parent or pediatrician may observe a young child frequently blinking, staring intensely for unusual periods, or repeatedly closing one eye at a time.
- There is a loss of communication skills and related cognitive abilities. A child with Rett syndrome who previously attained a degree of age-appropriate speech and language skills may begin to lose some of those abilities. In some children with the disorder, a more sudden and complete loss of speech and communication abilities may occur.
- There may be disinterest and diminished responses to environmental stimuli. As behavioral, physical, and cognitive changes begin to occur in a child with Rett syndrome, it often is observed that the child becomes less engaged and interested with people and objects. It may appear that the child is more interested in an internal world of perceptions and feelings than in interacting with her surroundings and other individuals in developmentally appropriate ways.
- Abnormal hand movements. As the disease progresses, children with Rett syndrome typically develop particular and very unusual hand movements, which may include clapping, rubbing, tapping, hand wringing, and hand squeezing.
- Abnormal behaviors. Parents and educators may observe very atypical behavioral patterns, including sudden, odd facial expressions, screaming for no apparent reason, and licking of the hands.
- Breathing problems that occur when a child is awake. A child with Rett syndrome may exhibit periods of breath holding , unusually rapid breathing, and forceful exhalation of air. These behaviors typically occur when a child is awake and not during sleep.

- Excessive irritability and related behavioral outbursts. Children with Rett syndrome may become increasingly agitated and irritable as they get older, often with no observable cause or as a result of minimal stressors in their environment. Periods of crying or screaming may begin suddenly and last for hours.
- Irregular heartbeat (dysrhythmia). Children and older individuals with Rett syndrome may have or develop cardiac problems involving dysrhythmia. Such conditions are serious and require appropriate medical interventions and monitoring.

ACQUIRED MEDICAL CAUSES OF INTELLECTUAL DISABILITIES

Pre- and postnatal exposure to alcohol, drugs, toxins, and certain infections can have very significant negative effects on brain development, and in many cases can result in an intellectual disability (American Psychiatric Association, 2013; Kerns, Don, Mateer, & Streissguth, 1997; Teeter & Semrud-Clikeman, 2007). The more common acquired prenatal causes (in utero) of intellectual disabilities include fetal alcohol syndrome and exposures to other drugs such as cocaine and heroin. The more common postnatal causes (during or after birth) include hypoxic ischemic injury (lack of oxygen during birth), traumatic brain injuries, exposure to toxins such as lead and mercury, and infections that affect the brain (American Psychiatric Association, 2013; O'Leary et al., 2013; Mattson & Vaurio, 2010).

Prenatal Exposure to Alcohol and Other Drugs

Fetal alcohol syndrome is one of the leading causes of preventable intellectual disabilities (National Organization on Fetal Alcohol Syndrome, 2014; American College of Obstetricians and Gynecologists, 2014). The syndrome causes brain damage and growth problems resulting from alcohol exposure of a fetus during the mother's pregnancy. The problems caused by fetal alcohol syndrome vary from child to child, but these defects are irreversible (National Organization on Fetal Alcohol Syndrome, 2014; O'Leary et al., 2013; Teeter & Semrud-Clikeman, 2007).

It is important for parents and educators to understand that not all individuals with fetal alcohol syndrome end up having a full intellectual disability. Virtually all children and adults with the syndrome, however, have varying combinations of cognitive deficits and related learning problems, along with various physical abnormalities and medical complications. Those concerns and effects can also occur with maternal use of other substances such as nicotine, cocaine, and heroin (American Psychiatric Association, 2013; National Organization on Fetal Alcohol Syndrome, 2014). Because it is not clear how much alcohol is safe to drink during pregnancy, most doctors recommend pregnant women avoid alcohol altogether (American College of Obstetricians and Gynecologists, 2014).

If a parent or early child educator suspects that a child has fetal alcohol syndrome, a pediatrician should be consulted as soon as possible, as early diagnosis and intervention may allow more positive outcomes.

ADAPTIVE BEHAVIORS

The term "adaptive behavior" refers to the collection of conceptual, social, and practical skills that have been learned by individuals in order to function in their everyday lives. Significant limitations in adaptive behavior impact a person's daily life and affect the ability to respond to a particular situation or to the environment. A significant deficit in one area impacts individual functioning enough to constitute a general deficit in adaptive behavior (AAIDD, 2014; Schalock, 2009). An overview of various adaptive behavior functions and skills are outlined in Table 3.1.

TABLE 3.1. Examples of Adaptive Behaviors

Conceptual skills: receptive and expressive language, reading and writing, money concepts, self-direction.

Social skills: interpersonal, responsibility, self-esteem, is not gullible or naive, follows rules, obeys laws, avoids victimization.

Practical skills: personal activities of daily living such as eating, dressing, mobility, and toileting; instrumental activities of daily living such as preparing meals, taking medication, using the telephone, managing money, using transportation, and doing housekeeping activities; occupational skills; maintaining a safe environment.

Is Intellectual Developmental Disorder the Same as Mental Retardation?

The diagnostic categories of intellectual disability and intellectual developmental disorder also refer to the same population of individuals who were previously and continue to be diagnosed under the term "mental retardation" in number, kind, level, type, and duration of disability. In addition, both diagnostic categories currently outlined by the AAIDD and the APA are consistent with recognizing the needs of people with diagnosed intellectual disabilities in regard to individualized services and supports.

EDUCATIONAL CONSIDERATIONS IN INDIVIDUALS WITH INTELLECTUAL DEVELOPMENTAL DISORDER

Educators working with individuals with intellectual developmental disorder may benefit from considering that such learners will likely have deficits in varying degrees and combinations in the areas of cognitive function listed in Table 3.2. It is also important for educators to consider that patterns and potentials for learning are unique to each individual with intellectual developmental disorder, based on the severity of the disability and individual cognitive strength and deficits (Schalock, 2009; Mervis & John, 2010).

TABLE 3.2 IMPORTANT ELEMENTS OF INTELLIGENCE

1. Abstract reasoning or thinking capabilities
2. The ability to solve problems through applied reasoning processes
3. Linguistic competence and related reasoning and understanding capacities
4. Visual-spatial processing and reasoning
5. Applied multiple functions of memory
6. Speed and efficiency of mental processing
7. The capacity to acquire knowledge
8. Fund of acquired general knowledge
9. Mathematical competence
10. Adaptation to one's environment
11. Applied creativity

Educators working with individuals recognized as having intellectual developmental disorder (as well as with learners with other neurodevelopmental disorders) may also benefit from understanding various historical and current theories of intelligence and models of learning based on neurodevelopmental constructs (AAIDD, 2014; Schalock, 2009).

HISTORICAL AND DEVELOPING CONCEPTS OF INTELLIGENCE

To facilitate the exploration of neurodevelopmental constructs and related learning and cognitive processes, an initial understanding of general intelligence and the related constructs of crystallized intelligence and fluid intelligence will provide a foundation for the understanding of applied and interactive cognitive facets of neurodevelopment. Those three categories of intelligence and cognition can indeed be conceptualized and understood as actual and specific neurodevelopmental constructs of cognitive processing and learning (Pennington, 2009).

Earlier views over the past century regarding the concepts of intelligence and human intellect were initially formulated with general assumptions that intelligence was a singular and unitary trait, like gender or height. Those views, however, evolved and developed over time into more complex theories of human cognitive functioning (Benjafield, 2005; Hergenhahn, 2009; Sattler, 2001; Sprinthall & Sprinthall, 1990). As such, in the beginning of the 20th century, it was theorized that human intelligence comprised two factors, an underlying general factor (g), and a series of very specific cognitive factors (s). That model of intelligence, proposed by British psychologist Charles Spearman, explained general intelligence (g) as the amount of overall mental energy that an individual possesses. Such general mental energy is involved with most types of more complicated mental activities such as applied reasoning functions, comprehension and understanding, higher-order language processing, and other related cognitive functions. In contrast, cognitive functions primarily mediated by specific cognitive factors (s) include less complex processes such as recall of information, speed of information processing (visual and verbal), and applied visual-motor abilities (Hergenhahn, 2009; Jensen, 1993, 1998; Sattler, 2001; Schultz & Schultz, 2008).

In the decades of related research on intelligence that followed, the various theoretical models that emerged generally emphasized a more general-factor (g) focus of intelligence, or a multiple-factor theory (s) of human intellect and functioning (Benjafield, 2005; Gardner, 1983; Lezak et al., 2004; Marx & Cronan-Hillix, 1987; Schultz & Schultz, 2008; Sprinthall & Sprinthall, 1990).

CRYSTALLIZED INTELLIGENCE AND FLUID INTELLIGENCE

If general intelligence (*g*) represents the overall mental energy of an individual that mediates more complex, integrated, and higher-order cognitive functions, are there other components of intelligence in addition to *g* and more specific (*s*) factors? In 1963, psychologist Raymond Cattell posited a theory of intelligence that included two additional general cognitive components, crystallized intelligence and fluid intelligence (Cattell, 1963; Sattler, 2001). With his colleague John Horn, Cattell's initial model of intelligence became well established over the next several decades and provided a foundation for subsequent theories that suggested other multidimensional models of intelligence (Benjafield, 2005; Carroll, 1997; Cattell & Horn, 1978; Dass et al., 1994; Hergenhahn, 2009; Horn, 1968, 1979, 1985; Horn & Noll, 1997; Schultz & Schultz, 2008; Sprinthall & Sprinthall, 1990).

Crystallized intelligence refers to cognitive processes and functions involving acquired knowledge and skills, while fluid intelligence describes the ability to problem solve using new information and tasks utilizing abstract mental thinking and mental agility (Cattell & Horn, 1978; Horn & Noll, 1997; Pennington, 2009; Sattler, 2001). Cognitive abilities involved in crystallized intelligence include acquired funds of both vocabulary and general knowledge, recall of previously learned and memorized information, and individual previous schematic knowledge and background experience.

Fluid intelligence is generally understood as involving one's mental flexibility, the ability to rapidly adapt and adjust to specific learning tasks and demands, the ability to resource abstract reasoning capabilities, and the capacity to quickly and effectively develop alternate cognitive response patterns and new thinking patterns (Ashcraft, 1989; Bachevalier et al., 1996; Cohen et al.,

1986; Horn, 1985; Horn & Noll, 1997; Lyon & Krasnegor, 1996; Matlin, 1989; Sattler, 2001).

Understood together in the contexts of both human intelligence and related learning processes, the cognitive components of general intelligence, crystallized intelligence, and fluid intelligence can also be considered as three essential and specific neurodevelopmental constructs of learning (Pennington, 2009).

Chapter 4

COMMUNICATION DISORDERS AND LANGUAGE DISABILITIES

Language and related expressions of communication, across many forms and modalities, are critical to the human experience and to our functioning in our day-to-day lives (Baker & Cantwell, 1987; Gualtieri et al., 1983; Kuder, 2003; Rourke & Fuerts, 1991). This is even more true across virtually all educational endeavors and settings. In regard to learning, teaching, and all areas of academic functioning, language is foundational in regard to the ability to process verbal and written information, to participate in classroom and course discussions, to establish effective working relationships with peers and teachers, and to understand, assimilate, and acquire new knowledge (Kuder, 2003; Levine, 2002a). An ability to understand and apply language concepts and principles, at many levels, is crucial to all areas of reading and written language, and to many areas of mathematical understanding and problem solving (Catts & Kamhi, 1999; Dawson & Guare, 2004; Emerson & Babtie, 2010; Henderson, 2012; Levine, 1998, 2002a, 2002b; Lyon & Krasnegor, 1996; Pennington, 2009; Sousa, 2008).

Given the importance of language in education as well as in so many areas of our lives, it is not surprising that difficulties, deficits, and developmental delays in any areas of language processing and understanding can have negative consequences for individuals educationally, socially, and vocationally (Baker & Cantwell, 1987; Cantwell & Baker, 1977; Mack & Warr-Leeper, 1992; Rourke & Fuerts, 1991). Quinn (2010) documented that three areas of speech and language impairments have been shown to cause disruption in a child's academic functioning and progress: (1) phonological awareness, (2) receptive language, and (3) expressive language. It has also been documented that the level of language development in preschool-age children is a very strong and important predictor of later acquisition of reading skills (Termine et al., 2007; Vargo, 2007).

LANGUAGE-BASED NEURODEVELOPMENTAL DISABILITIES

A language disability is a neurodevelopmental disorder characterized as developmental delays and deficits across various areas of language function and understanding, in the absence of other conditions such as intellectual impairment or severe psychiatric problems (Catts & Kamhi, 1999; Kamhi & Catts, 1989; Kuder, 2003; Quinn, 2010; Schmitt, Justice, & Pentimonti, 2013; Singer, 1990; Snowling & Hayiou-Thomas, 2010; Spafford & Grosser, 1996; Spreen et al., 1995; Stone, Silliman, Ehren, & Wallach, 2014; Swanson, Harris, & Graham, 2013). Language functions such as phonological processing provide the cognitive foundations for fundamental reading and spelling skills. Higher-order language functions such as semantic and pragmatic language support academic skills such as reading comprehension and written language. Developmental delays and deficits in any of those important language functions may significantly compromise language arts–related academic development. That is why dyslexic individuals, in addition to their reading difficulties, typically also have problems with spelling, expressive writing, word retrieval, and other facets of memory and learning

(Feifer & DeFina, 2000, 2002; Spafford & Grosser, 1996; Shay-witz, 2003).

Current clinical classifications of communication and language disorders, based on the American Psychiatric Association (2013) diagnostic codes include the subcategories of language disorder, speech sound disorder, childhood-onset fluency disorder, social (pragmatic) communication disorder, and unspecified communication disorder. Those specific categories of communication disorders can be understood within the contexts of the language functions and disabilities presented in this chapter.

Communication and language disorders include a range of language and related cognitive deficits that may include the form of language (phonology, syntax, morphology), the content of language (semantic language), and the function (pragmatics) of language (Catts & Kamhi, 1999; Hanson & Rogers, 2013; Kamhi & Catts, 1989; Quinn, 2010; Vargo, 2007, 2008). Children with language disorders, across all variations and levels of severity, typically share four common symptoms: (1) a deficiency or developmental delay in the quality of language that is learned, comprehended, and produced; (2) deficiencies in grammar understanding and applied usage; (3) developmentally delayed social communication skills; and (4) deficient nonverbal communication skills (Catts & Kamhi, 1999; Hanson & Rogers, 2013; Kamhi & Catts, 1989).

It has been estimated that approximately 2.4 million children in U.S. public schools experience various learning disabilities, which often involve primary or secondary language disabilities. Language processing disabilities can be considered within the context of neurodevelopmental disorders, which involve deficiencies and delays in neurological development and related cognitive functions (Spreen et al., 1995). It is well established that a significant number of children in the United States, estimated between 15% and 30%, suffer school failures that result from deficiencies in neurological development and related brain and learning dysfunctions (Hale & Fiorello, 2004; Spafford & Grosser, 1996; Levine, 2002a). Further, it has been noted that many students with various language-based and other neurodevelopmental disorders also experience ongoing difficulties in the social and emotional realms (Kuder, 2003; Rourke & Fuerst, 1992; Tanguay, 2006). Adolescents and adults with many neurodevelopmental disorders continue to experience challenges and difficulties in social and vocational areas of their lives. Not surprisingly, the ongoing difficulties that individuals with neurodevelopmental disorders struggle with across the developmental life span commonly involve eventual significant psychological and emotional problems such as depression, anxiety, and related behavioral issues (Rourke & Fuerst, 1991).

Language is not only a major communication modality critical to most human actions and endeavors, it is an essential component of many major counseling interventions (Corey, 2005; Corsini & Wedding, 2004). Cognitive-behavioral interventions, psychoanalytic therapies, and numerous other related insight-oriented therapies typically require (and assume) a developmentally appropriate command of functional and higher-order language capabilities (Seligman, 2006). Language-based neurodevelopmental disabilities, especially involving deficiencies in semantic and pragmatic language functions, can impact social, behavioral, and emotional functioning and development.

COMMON CHARACTERISTICS OF CHILDREN WITH LANGUAGE AND COMMUNICATION DISORDERS

Kuder (2003) outlined a range of common characteristics of children with language and communication disorders, within academic, social, cognitive, and behavioral domains (Table 4.1).

Research has also linked language disabilities with sensory-motor deficits (Quinn, 2010; Escalante-Mead, Minshew, & Sweeney, 2003), attention-deficit/hyperactivity disorder (Humphries, Koltun, Malone, & Roberts, 1994; Love & Thompson, 1998), visual-spatial processing (Nation, Marshall, & Altman, 2003), phonological processing (Breier et al., 2003; Quinn, 2010), memory and learning (Weismer, Plante, Jones, & Tamblin, 2005), executive functions (Hellend & Asbjoernsen, 2000), and speed and efficiency of information processing (Miller, Kail, Leonard, & Tomblin, 2001).

TABLE 4.1 CHARACTERISTICS OF CHILDREN WITH LANGUAGE AND COMMUNICATION DISORDERS

Cognitive Functioning
    Difficulty organizing information for recall
    Slow responding
    Inattentiveness

Academic Performance
    Reluctance to contribute to discussions
    Difficulty organizing ideas
    Difficulty recognizing phonemes
    Difficulty producing sounds
    Failure to follow directions
    Difficulty finding the right words for things

Social Interaction
    Reluctance to interact with other children
    Exclusion or rejection by other children
    Difficulty carrying on a conversation
    Problems negotiating rules for games

Behavior
  High level of frustration
  Frequent arguments
  Fighting with peers
  Withdrawing from interaction

It is not difficult to recognize how virtually all of the problematic common characteristics of language-disabled individuals presented by Kuder can significantly interfere with many areas of academic functioning and progress at all developmental levels, and may also manifest over time or contribute to emotional or behavior problems.

The following clinical case vignette may help elaborate how such difficulties can contribute to problems and delays in many academic areas.

CASE STUDY 4.1: ASHLEY

Ashley is a 15-year-old student in the ninth grade who has been struggling educationally over the past few years in all academic areas. Educational assessments several years earlier documented that Ashley has average-range overall academic abilities but delays in higher-order language abilities involving aspects of semantic and pragmatic knowledge, and written language deficits in applied knowledge of syntax and grammar structure.

Ashley has always had strong basic reading skills, including the ability to read and decode words with developmentally adequate fluency. As she has progressed through more advanced grade levels, however, Ashley has consistently presented notable delays in her reading comprehension abilities.

In addition, Ashley's performance on tests and in her

daily classroom activities is inconsistent. Her parents insist that Ashley studies consistently and for similar amounts of time at home for all of her tests, but nevertheless her test grades vary quite widely from week to week. Ashley herself states that when she is reading long passages while remaining reasonably focused, she often gets confused. Ashley also states that she frequently has difficulty recalling information that she "knows she learned and memorized" the night before a test.

Ashley underwent neuropsychological testing to obtain further information regarding her cognitive and learning strengths and weaknesses. That assessment confirmed a pattern of language-based learning deficits involving semantic and pragmatic language. The neuropsychological evaluation also revealed that Ashley has learning and memory deficits involving the ability to efficiently encode and (more notably) recall information consistently when she is required to do so. Ashley's current evaluation also indicated that she has executive function problems that affect her ability to self-regulate and self-monitor her learning processes and that also make it difficult for her to organize herself across many academic tasks, include lengthy and time-based writing assignments.

Based on the information obtained from the neuropsychological and educational evaluation, Ashley was provided with a range of special education interventions and accommodations, which included language instruction focused on enhancing higher-order language understanding and applications, specific instruction focused on organizational writing and reading comprehension, and instruction on effective studying strategies and executive function processes in wide educational contexts.

LANGUAGE DISABILITIES AND PSYCHOLOGICAL AND BEHAVIORAL DISORDERS

There is a large body of research documenting that a significant number of children with psychiatric, emotional, and behavioral disorders also have concurrent speech and language disabilities (Baker & Cantwell, 1987; Cantwell & Baker, 1977; Kuder, 2003; Vargo, 2008). A survey of those studies document that between 28% and 50% of children in psychiatric clinical setting and residential treatment programs have significant language disabilities (Cohen et al., 1989; Mack & Warr-Leeper, 1992; Gualtieri et al., 1983). Research also indicates similar associations between language disabilities and severely emotionally and behaviorally disordered children requiring special schooling (Trautman, Giddan, & Jurs, 1990), and even between less severely emotionally and behaviorally disordered children (Ruhl, Hughes, & Camarata, 1992).

CASE STUDY 4.2: AARON

Aaron is a 12-year-old sixth grader, with a well-established diagnosis of language-based learning disabilities, and more recent documentation of significant social language (pragmatic) deficits. Aaron continues to receive special education remedial interventions to address the academic deficits related to his disabilities.

Aaron was referred for individual counseling interventions to address his ongoing issues involving poor peer interactions, fighting in school, and mild depressive symptoms. In his initial counseling sessions, Aaron spoke of how other students in school would "make fun of him" and would "laugh at him." Aaron stated feelings of frustration and anger toward the teasing peers, especially because he frequently did not understand why they were laughing at him. Within the context of several initial counseling sessions, Aaron was able to describe in detail (his perceptions, of course) numerous past problematic peer interactions. It became evident that part of Aaron's confusion involved his lack of understanding of sarcasm and related ambiguous messages that the other students were actually communicating. It was also likely that Aaron's confusion and misunderstandings were also at times a source of amusement for some of the children.

Aaron's counselor integrated specific clinical goals in his treatment plan that targeted a better understanding and awareness of higher-order language processes related to the concepts of sarcasm and mixed verbal messages. Aaron was always allowed ample opportunities in his counseling sessions to give verbal feedback regarding his understanding of problematic events and peer interactions, as well as in regard to his understanding of clinical insights and concepts discussed in the therapeutic process.

With continued support and understanding that helped to facilitate a trusting clinical and therapeutic relationship, Aaron increased his developmentally appropriate expressive language and communication capabilities, resulting in a series of successful clinical interventions.

THE FIVE MAJOR LANGUAGE COMPONENTS

This section provides an in-depth overview of the major components and function of language and related educational considerations. A strong foundational understanding of the components and elements of language may provide educators across various academic disciplines with a better understanding of language disabilities, as well as how learning can be affected when various areas of language-based cognitions and functions are developmentally delayed or deficient.

Language can be understood as a complex and dynamic system

of symbols used for various processes of thinking, reasoning, and communication (Catts & Kamhi, 1999; Kuder, 2003; Stacey, 2003; Singer, 1990). Current understandings of language, based on contemporary societal rules and constructs, posit the following views and positions:

- Language evolves within specific social, cultural, and historical contexts.
- Language use and learning are determined by the interaction of biological, cognitive, environmental, and psychosocial factors.
- Language communication necessitates a comprehensive understanding of human interactions, such as nonverbal cues and sociocultural roles.
- Language is governed by at least five rule-based parameters and components.

The five rule-based parameters of language include phonology, morphology, syntax, semantics, and pragmatics.

The first three areas (phonology, morphology, and syntax) are critically relevant to reading and related academic processes, and are not of primary concern to most counseling situations (Rayner & Pollatsek, 1989; Wagner, Torgesen, & Rashotte, 1999; Vargo, 1992). Only a very brief review of those three areas of language is necessary for a counselor's understanding of those processes.

Phonology

Phonological processing refers to an individual's overall innate ability to hear, discriminate, recognize, and understand the various sound components in language (Vargo et al., 2004; Feifer & DeFina, 2000). Phonological awareness, the ability to hear and understand the sound-symbol correspondences of the printed page, is a critical component of early reading development (Rayner & Pollatsek, 1989). A reader's ability to decode words (sound out words using the rules of phonics) is strongly dependent upon the overall innate ability to hear, discriminate, recognize, and understand the various sound components in language (that is, the cognitive functions that involve phonological processing, memory, and awareness).

Morphology

What is also necessary for letter-sound combinations to make sense in a language is a set of rules that govern how words are made. Those rules are called morphological rules, and the related language component that governs those rules is known as morphology (Kuder, 2003; Rayner & Pollatsek, 1989; Stacey, 2003). Morphology, then, can be thought of as the study of words and how they are formed.

Morphemes are the smallest units of meaning in a language. An example of how words can be broken down into units of meaning can be found in the word "football." It can be broken down into two basic parts (morphemes), "foot" and "ball." As such, "football" has two morphological components that together comprise a single and uniquely meaningful word.

Syntax

Syntax can be understood as language at the sentence level. The established rules of syntax govern sentence organization, word order, and the relationship between words. Syntax regulates how words are combined into larger meaningful units of phrases and sentences, including grammatical structures such as noun and verb phrases (Akmajian et al., 1988; Greene & Coulson, 1995; Rayner & Pollatsek, 1989).

Syntax plays a critical role in the understanding and interpretation of grammar and subsequent language meaning (Singer,

1990). Given the depth and complexity of the role of syntax in language processing, it is easy to understand how neurodevelopmental deficiencies that affect syntactic processing and understanding can compromise language comprehension.

Semantics

Semantics is the aspect of language that governs the meanings of words and word combinations (Kuder, 2003; Rayner & Pollatsek, 1989; Singer, 1990). Consider the following sentence, which is linguistically appropriate in regard to the established rules of phonology, morphology, and syntax:

Empty buckets full of water laugh silently and with sadness.

The above sentence does not make sense according to the rules of semantics. The meanings of the words are contradictory and confusing. For instance, buckets cannot be both empty and full. Laughter is usually not silent and is typically not consistent with an emotional state characterized as sadness.

The English language, like many others, is rich with words that have multiple meanings, shades of meanings, and contextually driven meanings. For instance, the word "saw" can be both a noun and a verb, depending on the context of the sentence construct utilized. For example:

He saw the tool under the workbench.
He noticed the saw under the workbench.

In the first sentence, the word "saw" describes a process of seeing in the past tense. In the second sentence, the word "saw" describes a type of tool. To fully understand both sentences, a knowledge of the multiple meanings of "saw" is necessary, as well as an understanding of the technical and contextual meanings of the words in the sentence (e.g., an understanding of tools and workshops).

Students who are neurodevelopmentally delayed in aspects of semantic processing and understanding are at a disadvantage for acquiring a strong fund of vocabulary knowledge, that in turn helps to facilitate understanding and the acquisition of new knowledge through the reading process and other media (Spafford & Grosser, 1996). A semantically challenged individual in high school typically may have difficulty understanding many new words that are being read, and subsequently will not effectively learn and incorporate the new knowledge in the texts. Knowledge in subject areas such as math and science is often sequential and dependent on prior knowledge. Consequently, the student who has not grasped previous knowledge cannot learn additional concepts (Ashcraft, 1989; Matlin, 1989).

A good understanding of the components of semantic processing and awareness and the linguistic processes involved may allow counselors to work successfully with language-disabled clients. For instance, individuals with limited vocabulary knowledge may not always understand the words and verbal concepts presented to them, which may compromise an individual's receptive and expressive language processing abilities in daily life (Cohen et al., 1986).

Receptive language refers to an individual's capacity to understand (take in) language, while expressive language involves the production of language and related verbal expression skills (Greene & Coulson, 1995). Children with receptive language deficits can have difficulty following verbal directions and may have general verbal comprehension delays. Individuals with expressive language deficits may be immature in their language production skills and subsequent social language capacities, and they may have a limited capability to appropriately participate in many activities that involve language processes (Kuder, 2003).

Neurodevelopmental delays involving higher-order language

skills can also significantly compromise other communication modalities such as expressive writing, and may then subsequently involve long-term academic problems (Kuder, 2003; Spafford & Grosser, 1996; Stacey, 2003).

Pragmatic Language

The following sentence combinations (or variations of them) may be heard in the city of Boston during baseball season:

> Last night we saw the Sox in town. I had three large dogs and a couple of brews. We stayed all 12. When we left, the Pike was empty.

For those uninitiated in baseball terminologies and regional colloquialisms, and who may also be unfamiliar with contextual language familiar to the greater Boston area, the following translations of the above sentences may be helpful:

> Sentence translation 1: Last night I went to downtown Boston and saw the Boston Red Sox play a game of baseball against another team.
>
> Sentence translation 2: While I was at the game, I ordered and ate three rather large frankfurters on buns and drank two servings of beer.
>
> Sentence translation 3: We stayed for the entire game, which lasted 12 full innings.
>
> Sentence translation 4: When we left the game, we drove home on the Massachusetts Turnpike, which had a relatively light flow of traffic.

Residents of the Boston area, especially those who are Red Sox fans, would not need translations to fully understand the original sentences, because they would automatically employ context and related background knowledge to infer meaning (that is, fill in the blanks) that is not explicitly stated. The use of context and contextual knowledge is known as pragmatics (Catts & Kamhi, 1999; Singer, 1990). Pragmatics involves the use of language in social and environmental contexts. Listeners (and readers) who are not readily familiar with sociocultural references being utilized will simply not have an effective reference point to fill in the meanings that are not literally stated.

One simple example of the use of inferential thinking and understanding in language is the use of pronouns (Catts & Kamhi, 1999). The use of pronouns to reference subjects in a sentence (known as anaphora) is an inferential process that assumes the reader will make the appropriate subject-pronoun connections. For instance, the following series of sentences in a short paragraph form are grammatically correct, but linguistically redundant:

Gumby the cat lives with Erica's family. Gumby the cat is a beautiful cat with white fur. Gumby the cat likes to run around the house, and Gumby the cat takes lots of naps. The whole family loves Gumby the cat.

The constant repeated use (and literal reference) of "Gumby the cat" is linguistically cumbersome and not necessary. The following paragraph, utilizing the pronouns "he" and "him," (assuming Gumby is a male cat), is more appropriate:

Gumby the cat lives with Erica's family. He is a beautiful cat with white fur. Gumby likes to run around the house and take lots of naps. The whole family loves him.

It may be worthy of consideration for educators who are working with language processing–impaired students that such individuals may have problems with contextual language that may not be obvious or even recognized at all. Those problems can often underlie, or at least exacerbate, more obvious behavioral issues. For instance, a child or adolescent with specific difficulties in the use of pragmatic language may not easily recognize or understand sarcasm. Such a difficulty could result in that individual experiencing ongoing interpersonal conflicts with peers that could then result in dysfunctional behavioral episodes and feelings of poor self-esteem.

Chapter 5

ATTENTION-DEFICIT/ HYPERACTIVITY DISORDER

Attention, as a cognitive function, can be thought of as a neurodevelopmental construct that functions as the general manager of the brain. When attentional processes are effectively engaged in educational activities (or, in fact, any other activities or goal-directed behaviors) a child or older individual is able to efficiently maximize focus and deploy all potential cognitive and learning abilities and assets (Barkley, 1998; Levine, 2002a). The construct of attention enables an individual to appropriately and effectively filter out distractions, and to focus on the most important information in a learning activity long enough and with sufficient intensity to use and understand it well (Pennington, 2009; Willcutt, 2010).

Attention, in all of its components and processes, supports learning in numerous ways (D'Amato et al., 2005; Denckla et al., 2013; Levine, 2002a, 2002b). For example, when a student is able to concentrate effectively and consistently, that ability will enhance his or her memory for facts and can also support and strengthen the understanding of more complicated and higher-order language abilities. Components of attention also greatly facilitate the ability to effectively plan, to pace oneself, and to monitor and modify ongoing activities and behavioral and social functioning (Levine, 2002a; Lyon & Krasnegor, 2005).

Attention-deficit-hyperactivity disorder (ADHD) is one of the most common neurodevelopmental disorders (American Psychiatric Association, 2013; Barkley, 1998; Pennington, 2009). It is typically recognized during childhood and can continue through adolescence and adulthood (D'Amato et al., 2005). Surveys indicate that ADHD affects about 5% of children and about 2.5% of adults across most cultures (American Psychiatric Association, 2013). There is ample evidence to support that ADHD is a specific kind of brain dysfunction with strong genetic influences (Barkley, 1998; Pennington, 2009).

ADHD is characterized by age-inappropriate, chronic, and significant inattention and/or excessive motor restlessness and impulsivity (Hallowell & Ratey, 1994; Hanson & Rogers, 2013; Schweitzer, Pakyurek, & Dixon, 2013). Such behaviors and symptoms in an individual with ADHD typically occur in multiple settings that can result in difficulties and performance issues in many areas of life. For children and adolescents, those difficulties typically interfere with academic performance and functioning (Pennington, 2009). Adults with ADHD often have problems with work and other areas of functioning (Swanson et al., 2013).

SIGNS AND SYMPTOMS OF ADHD

Inattention, hyperactivity, and impulsivity are the key symptoms and behaviors of individuals with ADHD (Barkley, 1998; Hallowell & Ratey, 1994; Hanson & Rogers, 2013; Schweitzer et al., 2013). While it is normal for all children at various ages and developmental stages to be inattentive, hyperactive, or impulsive at times and to varying degrees, children and adults with ADHD typically have these behaviors at more severe levels and with more frequency than what is developmentally and behaviorally expected (Hallowell & Ratey, 1994). For a child to be diagnosed with ADHD, he or she must have diagnostically recognized symptoms for 6 or more months and to a degree that is greater than other children of the same age (American Psychiatric Association, 2013; Miller, 2010a).

Scientists are not sure what causes ADHD, although many studies suggest that genes play a large role in the disorder. In addition to genetics, research is also finding evidence of how environmental factors, brain injuries, nutrition, and the social environment might contribute to the disorder (Barkley, 1998; Pennington, 2009; Miller, 2010a; Teeter & Semrud-Clikeman, 2007; Yeates et al., 2010). Whatever the causes and etiologies, it is well established that the symptoms and resulting patterns of behavioral, emotional, educational, and social functioning can change across the life span of an individual who has the disorder and related cognitive and learning problems (D'Amato et al., 2005; Farran & Karmiloff-Smith, 2012; Miller, 2010a).

ADHD can occur together with other disorders, such as anxiety, depression, obsessive-compulsive disorder, bipolar disorder, and Tourette disorder. It is also important to note that the symptoms and behaviors of ADHD can also be components of psychiatric disorders that may be an individual's primary problem (Barkley, 1998; Hanson & Rogers, 2013; Schweitzer et al., 2013).

Treatment protocols for ADHD include medication interventions, instructions in behavioral and social skills management and training, behavior modification programming, and instructional counseling (Hale et al., 2010; Miller, 2010a; Pennington, 2009; Schweitzer et al., 2013).

A range of diagnostic symptoms and clusters of symptoms are used to support a diagnosis of ADHD and to help determine which subtype of the disorder is most prevalent. Those diagnostic guidelines involve various behavioral and cognitive dysfunctions that result in general and notable patterns of inattention, hyperactivity, and impulsiveness (see Table 5.1; American Psychiatric

Association, 2013; Barkley, 1998; D'Amato et al., 2005; Gold-berg, 2001; Hallowell & Ratey, 1994; Hanson & Rogers, 2013; Miller, 2010a; Pennington, 2009; Schweitzer et al., 2013).

TABLE 5.1 AHDH SUBTYPES
Inattention Problems

Individuals may be easily distracted, miss details, forget things, and frequently switch from one activity to another inappropriately.

Individuals may have difficulty focusing on one thing at developmentally appropriate levels.

Individuals may often become bored with a task after only a few minutes, unless they are doing something enjoyable to them.

Individuals may have difficulty focusing attention on organizing and completing a task or learning something new.

Individuals may have difficulty processing information at developmentally appropriate levels.

Individuals may often have difficulty following verbal directions.

Students often have trouble completing or turning in homework assignments, and may frequently lose things needed to complete tasks or activities.

Individuals may daydream excessively and may often seem to not listen when being spoken to.

Hyperactivity Problems

Individuals may have trouble sitting still during school and home activities at developmentally appropriate levels.

Children may be often observed to fidget and squirm in their seats excessively.

Children may appear to be constantly in motion and have difficulty doing quiet tasks or activities beyond developmentally appropriate expectations.

Children may dash around excessively (more than typical same-aged children) while often touching or playing with anything and everything in sight.

Impulsivity Problems

Individuals may often blurt out inappropriate comments, show their emotions without restraint, and act without regard for consequences.

Individuals may often inappropriately interrupt conversations or others' activities.

Children may present as very impatient and may often have difficulty waiting for things they want or waiting their turns in games.

THE ATTENTION CONTROL SYSTEM

The neurodevelopmental construct of attention actually has many components that occur and function in many ways when an individual's attentional capacities are activated during activities and behaviors (Teeter-Ellison, 2005). Levine (2002) posits a model of attention as consisting of three control systems: (1) the mental energy control system, (2) the processing control system, and (3) the production control system (Table 5.2). Based on this model, some children with ADHD experience problems with all of these attention systems, while others may show strengths and weaknesses in different systems. The following sections give a comprehensive overview of Levine's multidimensional model of attention.

TABLE 5.2 THE ATTENTION CONTROL SYSTEM

The Mental Energy Control System
Alertness control
  Mental effort control
  Consistency control
  Sleep and arousal control

The Processing Control System
Saliency determination control
  Depth and detail of processing
  Cognitive activation
  Focal maintenance
  Satisfaction control

The Production Control System
  Previewing
  Facilitation and inhibition
  Pacing/tempo
  Self-monitoring
  Reinforcement

Mental Energy Controls

The overall attention control system of mental energy regulates and distributes the energy supply needed for the brain to take in and interpret information and regulate behavior. If one thinks of the brain as a battery (the brain is in fact a bioelectrical system), then mental energy in this context can be thought of as the power source contained in the battery. Regardless of what metaphor one chooses to help to understand the concept, individuals whose mental energy is not used effectively may become chronically mentally fatigued when they try to concentrate, and may have other problems related to maintaining the brain energy needed for optimal learning and behavior.

There are four mental energy controls in this model. The first control is alertness, which can be understood as a state of mind in which an individual can effectively listen to and watch information being presented.

The second mental energy control is mental effort, which initiates and maintains the flow of mental energy required for an individual to initiate, effectively work on, and complete a task. Mental effort is particularly important when individuals are faced with tasks that may not be especially interesting or personally motivating. A parent, for instance, may believe that a child is not attentionally challenged because he or she can sit for hours completely focused on a favorite activity, such as a video game. It is important to understand, however, that when anyone is engaged in an activity that is intrinsically interesting or fun to that individual, that particular activity does not require an extensive regulation of attentional functions. In other words, you do not have to work hard to make yourself pay attention when you are doing something that is interesting or fun for you. However, one does have to marshal attentional resources when the task is less engaging and enjoyable, such as when a student needs to begin an academic task in school and maintain attention and focus at a developmentally appropriate level.

The third mental energy control is performance consistency, which works to ensure a reliable and predictable flow of mental energy over time and across tasks and activities. This model notes that individuals who have trouble with performance consistency may not have such problems all of the time, but consistency and predictability of performance can vary. One example of performance consistency deficits may be a child's inconsistent work production in class, observed over periods of time spanning hours to day and weeks.

The fourth mental energy control is sleep and arousal regulation, which affects an individual's ability to sleep well enough at night to be sufficiently alert during the day. Consider that children who are experiencing trouble with internal biological sleep and arousal mechanisms may find it difficult to get to sleep at night consistently, or they may often sleep poorly. Such difficulties may then result in trouble awakening in the morning and then persistent mental and physical fatigue throughout the day.

Processing Controls

The second attention control system is processing, which helps individuals in various activities and situations (including most learning contexts) to select and interpret incoming information. Levine's model supports the idea that individuals who have difficulty with processing controls may have a range of problems that can affect many learning and memory functions.

The model includes five processing controls. The first is saliency determination, which involves the ability to discriminate and select which incoming information is the most important to an individual. Consider that all humans are in one sense organisms that process information on many levels, and that much of that activity occurs below the threshold of conscious awareness. To function on all levels, we all are constantly screening information through many sensory systems that interactively involve the brain, the central nervous system, and related physical senses.

Individuals with saliency determination deficits may often be distracted by things in the environment that are not relevant to the present task or activity, while concurrently missing important information that is relevant. For example, a child with saliency determination problems is often distracted in class by noises and movements around him or her that most other students in the room are easily screening out of awareness to pay attention to a teacher who is speaking.

The second processing control is depth and detail of processing, which controls how intensely individuals can concentrate on highly specific information, and it enables learners to focus deeply enough to recognize and remember necessary details. For example, consider the amount of sustained mental energy that is involved in reading conceptually difficult material, or when significant amounts of information need to be learned and memorized.

The third processing control is cognitive activation, which helps learners most effectively connect new information to what has already been learned through prior knowledge and experience (such previously learned information is also known as schemas, or schematic knowledge). Based on this model, individuals who are less active processors than typical learners are less able to relate prior knowledge to new information. This model also posits that overactive processors of information may at times be cognitively distracted by too much prior knowledge that may not be relevant to the new incoming information, subsequently making it difficult to maintain focus.

The fourth processing control is focal maintenance, which allows an individual to effectively focus on information most important to a given task or activity for an appropriate amount of time. According to this model, for task completions to be most efficient given a learner's potentials, ideally there will be a good match between the duration of allotted attention and a given learning or activity goal.

The fifth processing control is satisfaction control, which involves an individual's ability to allocate enough attention to activities that are of moderate or low interest. Satisfaction control may involve similar and overlapping processes that are also involved in the mental energy control functions of this model.

Production Controls

The third attention control system in this model is production, which governs the output of functioning across many performance areas, including academic functioning and performance as well as many facets of behavioral and social functioning. Individuals with production control deficits may often present learning-related problems such as a tendency to work and do tasks too quickly and carelessly with minimal thought and planning.

There are five production controls in the model, beginning with the control functions of previewing. This control, when being implemented effectively, involves the ability to consider more than one action or response to an action, as well as the capacity to accurately anticipate the likely outcome of a particular choice or behavior. Individuals, for instance, who have difficulty with previewing controls may often plunge into activities and then react too quickly, with little or no regard for outcomes or consequences.

The second production control is facilitation and inhibition, which involves the ability to exercise emotional and behavioral restraint and not act or respond immediately to an event or situation. It also enables one to effectively consider multiple options, and to choose the best one before acting or starting on a task.

An example of dysregulation of facilitation and inhibition controls is when a child excessively and often inappropriately acts impulsively or perhaps constantly blurts out answers before being called upon in class.

The third production control is tempo/pacing. Effective regulation of this control results in performing tasks or activities at the most appropriate speed. A dysregulation may result in academic problems such as poor reading comprehension skills in otherwise skilled readers, as a result of skipping words and misreading multisyllabic words, as well as other reading processing mistakes.

The fourth production control in the model is self-monitoring, which allows individuals to effectively evaluate how they are doing while performing and after completing a task. Dysregulation of this control often makes it difficult for children and adults to check themselves while performing tasks and subsequently make corrective modifications and take action as needed to ensure successful completion of a task goal.

The fifth production control is reinforcement, which supports an ability to utilize previous experience to guide approaches to current tasks and behaviors. Consider an individual who repeatedly performs the same behaviors or actions despite repeated negative outcomes of those actions. Poor reinforcement controls in that individual may be making it difficult for him or her to change ineffective and perhaps even irrational behavioral patterns or task approaches.

ADHD AND EXECUTIVE FUNCTIONS

One of the least studied and most frequently overlooked contributors to academic and behavioral difficulties is learning problems recognized under the inclusive term executive functions. Difficulties in the executive functions are commonly associated with ADHD (Vargo et al., 2010; Yeates et al., 2010; Willcutt, 2010).

The executive functions are cognitive capabilities that are mediated primarily through the frontal lobes of the brain and directly involve a range of specific neurodevelopmental processes (Barkley, 1997; Dawson & Guare, 2004; Goldberg, 2001; Meltzer, 2007; Weyandt, 2005; Willcutt, 2010). Students with executive function deficits typically have neurobiologically based problems that can particularly affect learning processes involving planning, mental flexibility, organization, and self-monitoring of one's learning processes (Barkley, 1997; Levine, 1995; Meltzer & Krishnan, 2007). Research has clearly provided strong and consistent evidence that ADHD is a neurodevelopmental disorder that results from neurobiological and neurophysiological factors and dysfunctions (Castellanos et al., 2002; Hale et al., 2010; Miller, 2010a; Pennington, 2009).

Difficulties involving the regulation of attentional processes, such as attention-deficit disorder (ADD) or ADHD, are common correlates with executive dysfunctions (Barkley, 1997; Goldberg, 2001). As such, individuals diagnosed with attentional disorders commonly exhibit many of the learning problems associated with developmentally delayed executive skills. Educators may frame those associations within an understanding that ADD and ADHD most typically involve a range of learning problems in addition to developmentally delayed attentional capabilities.

Executive Functions Defined

The executive functions involve a range of cognitive skills and capabilities that allow one to coordinate and integrate existing knowledge and skills in order to pursue particular goals. The executive functions are not primarily concerned with what one actually knows and can do. However, they are primarily related to how and whether one is able to use knowledge and skills in goal-directed ways.

The executive functions include such crucial multifaceted learning skill sets as goal formulation and planning, the generation and organization of learning strategies, attentional control, the generation and flexible shifting of mental sets, the inhibition of impulsive responses, and the regulation and monitoring of one's own performance (Barkley, 1997; Dawson & Guare, 2004; Goldberg, 2001). Other executive-based cognitive and learning functions and subfunctions that are individually and interactively crucial to most successful learning processes and tasks are as follows:

1. The ability to understand and follow information sequentially
2. The ability to prioritize important information when learning
3. The ability to effectively organize, process, encode, and retrieve information
4. The ability to self-initiate tasks (e.g., how to begin a project)
5. The ability to inhibit impulsive responses and behaviors
6. The ability to shift cognitive sets between learning activities

Specific Observable Symptoms and Traits of Poor Executive Functioning

Students with executive dysfunctions often present a range of learning and even behavioral problems that can and often do interfere with academic functioning and progress (Barkley, 1997). Some of those symptoms and traits include, but are not limited to:

1. Difficulties following and understanding verbal information at developmentally appropriate levels
2. Difficulties following multiple-step directions
3. Inconsistent academic performance
4. Immature emotional controls

5. Low frustration tolerance
6. Selective attention

Some specific examples of educational difficulties related to executive dysfunctions (and specific questions that educators can ask) include the following:

- Goal-directed behaviors and persistence: At a developmentally appropriate level, can a student follow through with an academic task (or other tasks) without being easily distracted or drawn to other activities before task completion?
- Task initiation: At a developmentally appropriate level, can a specific student understand how to begin a multifaceted learning task? Can that student then organizationally follow through with an effective planned sequence to complete that task? For instance, a lengthy term paper or writing project requires beginning with a plan of how to first research and acquire information, then sequentially organize that information, and then develop a completed written work assimilating and presenting that information and newly acquired knowledge.
- Mental flexibility: At a developmentally appropriate level, can a student shift attention from one task activity to another? Can a student in the classroom (or in other environments) adjust successfully to unexpected changes in routine or expectations?
- Self-regulation of affect: At a developmentally appropriate level, can a student manage and control emotions while practicing effective goal-directed and on-task behaviors?
- Response inhibition: At a developmentally appropriate level, can a student inhibit impulsive responses or behaviors? For instance, a child with executive dysfunctions may be unable to control his verbal responses in class if he frequently blurts out answers before raising his hand.

CASE STUDY 5.1: JASON

Jason is a 12-year-old sixth grader with a previous diagnosis of ADHD. Jason has been prescribed medications to address his attentional difficulties for the past several years, with reported reasonable success. Despite his improved ability to stay focused and on-task in the classroom, however, Jason's academic performance remains inconsistent and well below expectations consistent with his previously assessed intellectual capabilities. Jason remains very disorganized in school, especially in regard to his ability to keep track of daily homework and more long-term homework assignments. He has particular difficulty with expressive writing, despite his obvious general language and especially expressive language strengths. His parents report that Jason studies hard before a test, but that his ability to recall information that he apparently has learned is inconsistent when he is actually tested.

Jason's difficulties were assessed and better understood by his teachers and parents within the context of multiple executive dysfunctions. His teachers worked as a team to develop and implement consistent and specific educational accommodations across all of his classroom and academic environments.

Jason's parents were active partners with his teachers and aided in their son's organizational management of assignments and academic tasks between school and home. Jason also began to receive specific remedial interventions in expressive writing, with a strong focus on the organizational process of writing.

After several months of combined and consistent educational remediations and specific remedial interventions, Jason's overall academic performance (and his academic grades) improved significantly.

Developmental Considerations

The physiological development of the brain and related cognitive processing capacities directly relate to how executive function disorders can extend and manifest differently across the life cycle, from infancy through adulthood (Bronson, 2000; Dawson & Guare, 2004; Teeter & Semrud-Clikeman, 1997). It is crucial for educators to understand such developmental and related learning processes when teaching children and adolescents of various ages and grade levels. For instance, a student who leaves grammar school for middle school needs to access higher levels of executive and related organizational management skills, given the expanded structures and schedules of the upper grade levels. While most students typically find the elementary–middle school transition challenging, children with executive dysfunctions may be more easily overwhelmed by the new academic and developmental expectations of the higher grades (Dawson & Guare, 2004).

Neurodevelopmental Considerations

There is a direct relationship between physical brain development and maturation, and a child's levels of cognitive and executive functioning (Barkley, 2007; Berninger & Richards, 2002; Baron, Fennel, & Voeller, 1995; Batchelor & Dean, 1996; Dawson & Guare, 2004; Levine, 1995; Rourke, Bakker, Fisk, & Strang, 1983; Spreen et al., 1995; Teeter & Semrud-Clikeman, 1997). Physical brain development and maturation continue from very early childhood into late adolescence and very early adulthood, which includes the continuing maturation of the frontal lobes and prefrontal cortex areas of the brain (Kolb & Wishaw, 1990; Spreen et al., 1995; Teeter & Semrud-Clikeman, 1997). It is generally agreed upon by neuroscientific researchers that the human frontal brain systems, including the frontal/prefrontal cortex and adjacent areas, are the primary brain structures that correlate with most cognitive processes involving the executive functions (Barkley, 2007; Bronson, 2000; Dawson & Guare, 2004; Teeter & Semrud-Clikeman, 1997). Research indicates that the brain structures that underlie the executive functions are quite complex and also include connections between other brain regions, such as the subcortical regions (Durston, 2003; Fletcher, 1996; Weyandt, 2005).

Levine (1995) outlined a range of general and subsequent specific learning difficulties related to executive dysfunctions and cognitive deficits and delays. Levine refers to general difficulties as themes and related specific difficulties as observable phenomena. The latter category provides a sound framework for educators to utilize to monitor observable learning issues and likely related underlying cognitive problems. An outline of Levine's framework of neurodevelopmental themes and related observable phenomena is as follows:

Themes	Observable Phenomena
Weak attentional controls	Weak mental energy controls
	Weak information-processing controls
	Weak work production controls
Reduced remembering	Problems with short-term memory functions
	Insufficient active working memory
	Incomplete consolidation in long-term memory
	Reduces access to long-term memory stores
Chronic misunderstanding	Weak language processing
	Incomplete language formation

Themes	Observable Phenomena
	Developmentally delayed or weak visual processing
	Developmentally delayed or weak data processing
	Small chunk-size capacity (amounts of information)
	Excessive top-down or bottom-up processing
Deficient output	Weak language production
	Developmentally delayed fine-motor performance
	Persistent organizational failure
	Problems with general problem solving and strategies
Delayed skill acquisition	Developmentally slow reading development
	Inaccurate or poor spelling patterns
	Developmentally poor or impeded written output
	Developmentally poor or impeded math abilities
Poor behavioral adaptation	School-related sadness or dissatisfaction
	Noncompliant behaviors or behavioral acting out
	Poor or lost motivation
	Poor socialization abilities
	Developmentally inappropriate bodily preoccupations

Levine's framework of neurodevelopmental themes and observable phenomena outlines a wide range of often concurrent and interactive learning and academic problems and deficits that typically correlate with executive dysfunctions and related neurocognitive deficits. Executive dysfunctions and cognitive organizational difficulties often manifest as difficulties regulating and controlling cognitive and attentional functions, deficient learning capabilities (which often include deficient encoding and retrieval capacities), and delayed specific academic skills such as reading comprehension and expressive writing (Berninger & Richards, 2002; Mayer, 1998; Levine, 1995).

Chapter 6

AUTISM SPECTRUM DISORDER

Autism spectrum disorder (ASD) is a complex neurodevelopmental disorder that is estimated to occur today in approximately 1 out of 150 children, occurs four times more commonly in males, and has strong genetic components (American Psychiatric Association, 2013; Bauman & Kemper, 1994; Goldstein & Reynolds, 2011; Lang, 2010; National Institute of Neurological Disorders and Stroke, 2013; Ozonoff, 2010; Pennington, 2009). While ASD occurs across a spectrum of degrees and variations of clinical profiles, three core deficits in functioning and developmental processes are common to the disorder: (1) deficiencies in social interactions and functioning based on expected typical developmental levels, (2) deficits and developmental delays in functional language and communication skills, and (3) restricted areas of personal interest and often observable patterns of stereotypical behaviors (Durand, 2014; Frith, 2008; Hanson & Rogers, 2012; Lang, 2010; Rogers et al., 2013). While the severity and symptomatic patterns of ASD are quite variable, the interrelated symptoms of the disorder will always have a significant effect on an individual's performance and functioning across all areas of life (Frith, 2008; Lang, 2010; Rogers, Ozonoff, 2010; Ozonoff & Hansen, 2013).

Children with ASD are often first evaluated and recognized in early childhood, typically during preschool years. Presenting symptoms that often raise concerns and precipitate evaluation may include delayed speech and language functions, poor or unusual interpersonal and social interactions, repetitive odd vocal patterns and productions, notable nonsocial attachments (e.g., unusual focus on objects or playthings), and unusual responses to sensory stimuli such as sounds, lights, and many other environmental influences (Corbette & Schulte, 2011; Frith, 2008; Lang, 2010; Miller, 2010a).

Durand (2014) outlined characteristics of ASD that are consistent with current diagnostic components and research into this neurodevelopmental disability. He emphasized two major general characteristics of ASD that are outlined in the *Diagnostic and Statistical Manual of Mental Disorders*, fifth edition: (a) impairments in social communication and interaction; and (b) restricted behaviors, interests, and activities. For a diagnosis of ASD to be established, an individual must exhibit notable difficulties in areas of both communication and socialization, as well as behavioral functioning. There must also be evidence that an individual with a symptomatic profile consistent with ASD also has a limited ability to function adequately in virtually all social contexts. In fact, a consistent defining characteristic of ASD across current research and diagnostic definitions is that all noted problematic behaviors and characteristics must be at a level of significant limitations and impairments in the ability of an individual to function in most or all levels of society (American Psychiatric Association, 2013; Atwood, 2008; DeOrnellas, Hood, & Novales, 2010; Frith, 2008; Pennington, 2009).

COMMUNICATION PROBLEMS ASSOCIATED WITH AUTISM SPECTRUM DISORDER

All three of the following general types of communication difficulty need to be present in an individual to support a diagnosis of ASD (Bauminger-Zviely, 2013; Buron & Wolfberg, 2008; Durand 2014; Lang, 2010):

- Difficulties with social reciprocity: An individual with ASD, according to the severity of the disorder, will have varying degrees of difficulty with back-and-forth conversations, and a general inability to communicate with others about common interests or situations (Buron & Wolfberg, 2008; Tager-Flusberg & Anderson, 1991).

- Difficulties with nonverbal communication: Communication with others includes many aspects of nonverbal communication. Physical gestures, facial expressions, tone and prosody of voice, and other often subtle nonverbal actions are all involved in effective communication processes. An individual with ASD, according to the severity of the disorder, may lack accurate understanding or may not even be aware of many nonverbal communication signals, cues, and messages, with subsequent difficulties and dysfunctions in communications with others. Some individuals with ASD may have a complete lack of interest in developing and maintaining friendships and relationships with others.

- Difficulties in creating or maintaining relationships with others: An individual with ASD, according to the severity of the disorder, will have varying degrees of difficulty being comfortable in many social situations and contexts, and may also have related difficulties navigating social interactions and activities between individuals and groups.

RESTRICTED OR REPETITIVE PATTERNS OF BEHAVIORS, ACTIVITIES, OR INTERESTS

At least two of the following characteristics should be present in an individual to support a diagnosis of ASD (American Psychiatric Association, 2013; Durand, 2014; Lang, 2010; Ozonoff, 2010; Rogers et al., 2013):

- Varying degrees of problems with aspects of physical speech production and motor movements (Myles & Simpson, 1998; Rogers et al., 2013).
- Excessive dependence on routines and high sensitivity to changes in established routines or the environment in general, and can include intense focus on inappropriate items (Durand, 2014; Matson & Nebel-Schwalm, 2007; Miller, 2010a).
- Exceptional and consistent strong fixations on certain topics or objects (DeOrnellas et al., 2010; Durand, 2014; Frith, 2008).
- Unusual or problematic responses to various sensory input (Hanson & Rogers, 2012; Lang, 2010; Minshew & Williams, 2008), such as hyperreactive to textures (e.g., certain clothing fabrics), loud noises, odors (e.g., perfumes or colognes), or bright lights.

It is important to emphasize again that the symptoms of ASD fall on a continuum, ranging from mild to severe. This continuum allows clinicians to account for the variations in symptoms and behaviors among individuals. As such, when working with individuals with ASD, it may be helpful to consider that each individual with the disorder will present symptoms and behaviors in unique ways according to individual strengths and weaknesses (Lang, 2010; Pennington, 2009).

OTHER CONDITIONS THAT MAY COEXIST WITH AUTISM SPECTRUM DISORDER

There are other medical and psychological conditions that an individual with ASD may also have, especially older children, adolescents, and adults (Bolton et al., 2011; Dykens & Lense, 2011; Ivarsson & Melin, 2008; Ozonoff, 2010; Rogers et al., 2013). The coexistence of two or more forms of psychopathology in one individual is also referred to as comorbidity (Matson & Nebel-Schwalm, 2007). Comorbid clinical concerns should also be investigated when a diagnosis of ASD is being considered, either to rule out other possible medical or clinical explanations for presenting symptoms or to identify other concurrent issues and problems that will also need to be addressed in any treatment and educational plan. Some additional clinical or medical issues that may be a component of ASD include intellectual disability, ADHD, mood disorders such as depression and anxiety, obsessive-compulsive disorder, epilepsy, motor skill deficits, language deficits, executive function deficits, learning and memory deficits (Ozonoff, Pennington, & Rogers, 1991), sleep disorders, gastrointestinal problems, and eating and feeding problems (Bolton et al., 2011; Durand, 2013; Dykens & Lense, 2011; Filipek, 2005; Ivarsson & Melin, 2008; Ledford & Gast, 2006; Matson & Nebel-Schwalm, 2007; Noterdaeme, Amorosa, Mildenberger, Sitter, & Minnow, 2001; Ozonoff, 2010; Ozonoff et al., 1991; Rogers et al., 2013; Simonoff et al., 2008; Tuchman, 2011; Wang, Tancredi, & Thomas, 2011).

EDUCATIONAL CONSIDERATIONS

Characteristic patterns of strengths and weaknesses in various areas of academic functioning have been researched and noted in individuals with ASD (DeOrnellas et al., 2010; Mayes & Calhoun, 2003; Minshew & Williams, 2008; O'Connor & Klein, 2004; Ozonoff, 2010). While individuals with more severe degrees and patterns of the disorder and concurrent significant impairments of general intellectual capacities may understandably present multiple areas of academic difficulties and delays, students with higher-functioning ASD may have patterns of cognitive and related academic strengths. For instance, higher-functioning individuals with ASD may have strong fundamental reading skills at the word level (e.g., word identification, decoding, and automaticity), but may concurrently have marked delay in reading comprehension abilities due to disorder-related cognitive and language deficits. Students with higher-functioning ASD typically also have academic delays in written language and general language arts (Mayes & Calhoun, 2003; Tager-Flusberg & Anderson, 1991).

Minshew and Williams (2008) proposed understanding ASD as a disorder of information processing, grounded in current neuropsychological and neuroimaging research. They outlined an overview of typical patterns of cognitive strengths and weaknesses that support or hinder academic functioning in individuals with high-functioning ASD (Table 6.1).

TABLE 6.1 HIGH-FUNCTIONING AUTISM: STRENGTHS AND DEFICITS

Intact or Enhanced Abilities	Cognitive Weaknesses
Attention	Complex motor functions
Sensory perception	Complex memory functions
Elementary motor functions	Complex language
Simple memory functions	Concept formation
Formal language	Face recognition
Rule learning	
Visuospatial processing	

Minshew and Williams (2008) offered the following educational considerations for student with ASD, with additional suggestions based on other sources and areas of research (Buron & Wolfberg, 2008; DeOrnellas & Schulte, 2011; Goldstein & Reynolds, 2011; Hobsen, 2012; Lang, 2010; Mayes & Calhoun, 2003; Miller, 2010; Myles & Simpson, 1998; Noterdaeme et al., 2001; O'Connor & Klein, 2004; Pennington, 2009; Pennington & Ozonoff, 1996; Tager-Flusberg & Anderson, 1991; Yeates et al., 2010).

Students with ASD, across all levels of the disorder, typically have difficulties processing large amounts of information efficiently. Thus, information presented to such students may consistently need to be reduced to manageable amounts, with an emphasis on conceptual content rather than many facts and details.

Students with ASD process language differently than typically developing learners. Thus, information verbally presented to learners with ASD may consistently need to be very clear, concise, and more slowly given according to the needs of each individual learner. Thematic teaching, whereby a topic of interest for a learner is used as a medium for teaching academic content information, may be of great value to students with ASD.

Students with ASD typically have problems organizing material, information, processes, and schedules, and related difficulties in executive functions that support those abilities. Thus, learners across the spectrum may benefit from having a specific staff contact at the end of each school day to aid in organization of homework and assignments and to review proceedings of the day. In addition, it may benefit learners on the ASD spectrum to be presented new information visually and verbally, along with previews of main ideas and concepts. Graphic organizers and semantic maps visually presenting main ideas and relationships can be helpful to all students, but particularly to anyone with organizational difficulties, such as learners with ASD. The utilization of repetition and structured learning routines across academic tasks and content areas may be of great benefitto facilitate and consolidate learning.

Many of the common difficulties in individuals with high-functioning autism in the areas of language processing and understanding may also manifest as deficits in reading comprehension, written language, and applied mathematics (Buron & Wolfberg, 2008; Hobsen, 2012; Minshew & Williams, 2008; O'Connor & Klein, 2004). It is well established that developmental delays and deficits in areas of higher-order language processing and understanding can adversely affect academic performance and development in areas of language arts at the levels of comprehension, understanding, and communication (Catts & Kamhi, 1999; Feifer & DeFina, 2000, 2002; Kamhi & Catts, 1989; Kuder, 2003; Rayner & Pollatsek, 1989; Singer, 1990; Spafford & Grosser, 1995). For instance, difficulties in understanding semantic language can affect a reader's ability to effectively use inferencing capabilities to facilitate text comprehension (Catts & Kamhi, 1999; Rayner & Pollatsek, 1989). Problems with organization of thinking and processing can compromise an individual's ability to effectively develop and construct writing tasks and projects (Feifer & DeFina, 2002). Problems with higher-order language and concept formation can interfere with a learner's ability to solve conceptually based math problems (Emerson & Babtie, 2010; Henderson, 2012; Sousa, 2008).

CASE STUDY 6:1 TYLER

Tyler is a 6 year old boy who lives with a biological parent and two older siblings (ages 8 and 11), and attends kindergarten in the public school system of his community. He was referred by his school system and his parents for intellectual/cognitive, developmental language, and occupational therapy evaluations because of concerns in school and at home regarding Tyler's cognitive, language, and social functioning and development. Further concerns that prompted an assessment process for Tyler included a long history for him of language and developmental delays and patterns of atypical behaviors. Those concerns, noted by his parents since approximately the ages of one and two and throughout his preschool years, have been repeatedly shared and initially addressed by Tyler's pediatrician and several specialists involved in early language development and remediation.

Tyler's documented early developmental history documented no pre-natal or birth related concerns. After a full-term pregnancy and natural birth with no post-natal complications, Tyler was considered by his pediatrician and his parents to be a healthy infant with no apparent medical concerns or conditions. By age one, however, Tyler's parents noted that their son did not seem to respond to his environment and others as well as his parents and siblings in many of the ways that their older children did at that age. For instance, when his parents held him and talked as a baby, Tyler typically appeared to be unable to maintain eye contact for more than a few seconds, and at times he would not make eye contact at all. Tyler's parents reported that when he was held as a baby and even as a very young toddler, he would often appear to be uncomfortable and emotionally unresponsive, and would sometimes even physically stiffen his body in response to physical contact such as a hug. Tyler did play with toys, but he usually remained interested in several specific toys that he would focus on for longer periods of time. His parents long observed that as a toddler and preschooler, Tyler always seemed most comfortable playing alone and amusing himself with favorite toys and objects. He often seemed, reported his parents, like he was "in a world all his own".

Right after his first birthday, Tyler's parents brought him to his pediatrician to address concerns they had regarding their son having possible hearing deficits because he rarely responded when they called him by name. Tyler's hearing, however, was determined to be not impaired. By the beginning of his second year, Tyler was not presenting any functional expressive language skills even close to developmental norms. He did begin at that age to often repeat words over again for seemingly no reason, and at times he would repeatedly verbalize short phrases that he heard from television commercials or from adults speaking. As Tyler grew older, from ages three to five, his functional communication skills did increase, but at a rate much slower than expected developmental levels and norms.

During the ages of four and five, Tyler began to exhibit frequent rocking behaviors, and was more infrequently observed to wave his hands in the air in a sustained manner for no apparent reason. Also during that age period, his parents observed that Tyler at times would seem to react adversely to various smells, tastes, and sounds that seemingly should not have bothered him.

At age five, his parents enrolled Tyler several days a week for nine months in a pre-school program, with the primary goal of offering him opportunities to better develop his interpersonal and socialization skills. While Tyler's functional communication skills during that time were developed enough so that he could verbalize simple questions and requests (e.g., expressing his need to toilet or that he was hungry), it was noted by the staff in his program that Tyler's ability to interact with other children his age was very developmentally limited. While he was capable of interacting with a peer or with several children in the context of shared participation of activities that he enjoyed, Tyler more typically preferred to play or pursue activities by himself. He was also observed when he was with other children to not be aware of even basic personal space issues. For instance, at times Tyler would speak to another child while standing literally nose-to nose with him or her), and he often would speak in unusual tones or with excessive and inappropriate levels of volume.

Tyler's parents hoped that his preschool experiences would help him to develop more age typical communication and socialization skills, and they were also hopeful that perhaps he was developmentally simply a "late bloomer". When he began kindergarten, however, his teacher quickly became concerned about Tyler's very obvious social and functional communication deficits. According to his teacher, Tyler did not have too much difficulty following the usual routines across an entire school day. In fact, he quickly learned and responded well to the established daily routines, such as knowing that "snack time" everyday followed the morning reading group, and that recess time followed lunch. However, when those routines were disrupted or even slightly deviated from, Tyler would almost always become visibly upset and at times even responded with episodes of tantrum behaviors until he could be calmed down.

The cognitive component of Tyler's evaluation that was requested by his kindergarten teacher and subsequently by the school system's special education department was inconclusive. Tyler engaged in some of the language and non-language tasks presented to him, but apparently did not understand or could not respond to other others. He could, for instance, name various pictures of age appropriate pictures presented to him, and he was able to respond to simple question, such as, "what can you wear on your head when it rains?" When he was presented with verbal and perceptual questions and tasks that required higher developmental levels of reasoning and understanding, Tyler was not able to accurately respond for his age or engage at all. As a result, standardized assessments of Tyler's overall levels of intellectual functioning were unattainable, although it was noted that his cognitive functions in most assessed areas overall appeared to fall within ranges of a child with an intellectual disability.

The occupational therapy evaluation conducted on Tyler indicated that he was moderately developmentally delayed in various fine-motor and gross motor functions. Most of those assessed delays were for the most part not severe and notable obvious in regard to Tyler's observable general physical capabilities such as his ability to walk and run or to manipulate objects while holding them. However, the degree of the developmental delays noted from the occupational therapy assessment were noted by the examiner to be likely significant enough to interfere with fine-motor related tasks such as hand writing, and using painting tools and scissors in craft related activities. It was also noted that Tyler's assessed moderate gross motor delays, without remedial interventions, could result in problems involving the development of general physical activities and skills, such as early physical education activities and learning how to ride a bicycle.

The school based assessment also included the use of autism rating scales on Tyler that were completed separately by both of his parents and his teacher. Based on the cumulative information from those scales and recent observations during his preschool and kindergarten experiences, along with a full consideration of his prior developmental history, Tyler was diagnosed as having Autism Spectrum Disorder.

Based on the information obtained from his assessment processes, an Individualized Educational Plan (IEP) was developed for Tyler, and implemented throughout all aspects of his educational programming. Some of the information included in Tyler's IEP, based on his diagnosis of Autism Spectrum Disorder, included the following:

It was determined by all participants on his educational team that Tyler's educational programming would occur as much as possible in mainstream classes with all necessary staff and supports. As such Tyler was able to interact and assimilate with typically developing peers as much as possible and when determined most appropriate.

A specialized curriculum and broad program of studies,

with scope and sequence of information structured specifically for him was developed for Tyler that encompassed his academic and educational needs involving the progressive acquisition of academic skills sets and abilities to his ultimate full capabilities. For instance, ongoing individual and small-group instructions for basic reading and fundamental math occurred daily for Tyler with other students who had similar educational and clinical needs as him.

Tyler's initial academic skills in all basic content areas were initially assessed to provide a baseline that would allow for accurate measurement and monitoring of progress across academic areas in his educational programming. Once academic baselines were established, Tyler's educational team developed individualized assessment measures and timelines appropriate to his unique educational needs to consistently monitor all areas of educational progress.

Tyler's Individual Educational Plan included a strong component of remedial language teaching and instructions, which occurred several times a week in a small group of no more than four students who also had similar profiles and challenges educationally and clinically similar to him. Those focus of the language instructions included addressing language deficits common to early elementary aged school children and in fact most individuals with the disorder across the life span. More specifically, Tyler was progressively introduced to and then extensively allowed to practice higher-order language understandings and concepts, focusing on beginning understandings of linguistic areas such as literal vs. non-literal language and communication, the understanding and application of established rules and understandings of social communication, pragmatic language concepts and utilizations, metaphors (e.g., for a young child, learning to understand how a story can teach a lesson), and even sarcasm in communication and written language contexts. Tyler's language instructions initially focused on the learning and understanding of social-cognitive precursors that are critical to early language acquisition, and then following with systematic progression of teaching focusing on increasing understanding of language content and meanings. There was also a strong component of training in the language components of Tyler's Individual Educational Plan that included expressive verbal language, enhanced receptive language capabilities, and nonverbal communication understandings and skills.

All of the language instructions that Tyler received and would continue to receive as he progressed through higher grade levels were taught and practiced in the contexts of social communication and interpersonal interactions, as well as in academic contexts. For instance, understanding how even simple sentences and readings at early elementary grade levels can require a young reader to understand and utilize a fundamental awareness of context and inferences while reading to glean intended and accurate understanding. Tyler was provided with a weekly social skills group with a consistent small group of students with educational and clinical issues similar to his own. Many of the concepts that he was taught in his remedial language instructions were integrated and practiced in the social skills group activities.

Tyler's educational programming included individual occupational therapy training sessions several times per week focusing on him progressively developing stronger fine-motor and gross-motor skills.

Tyler's Individualized Educational Plan allowed for his increased engagement and flexibility in developmentally appropriate tasks and play, both individually and in the context of interactions with typically developing peers. To help him to consistently and effectively attend to his environments, Tyler's school system developed for him an individualized behavior modification program that was used throughout all of his school day. Tyler's behavioral plan was developed by a board certified applied behavioral analysis specialist and implemented continuously in school by the staff supporting him in all of his classes that were trained in the necessary procedures required of the behavioral program.

Tyler's school system provided consistent communication protocols and procedures with his parents, to ensure that all of his progress was continuously communicated with his parents and that a consistency of programming and services was established and continued between school and home.

ASPERGER'S DISORDER

Asperger's disorder, also called Asperger's syndrome, is a type of developmental disorder involving delays in the development of many basic skills, most notably the ability to socialize with others and to communicate effectively. The disorder also commonly involves restrictive, repetitive, and stereotyped patterns of behavior (Ghaziuddin, 2005; Myles & Simpson, 1998).

Previous to the establishment of current diagnostic criteria for ASD in the *Diagnostic and Statistical Manual of Mental Disorders*, fifth edition (American Psychiatric Association, 2013), the diagnostic category of Asperger's disorder in the *DSM-IV-TR* was included with the diagnosis of autistic disorder, under the more general category of pervasive developmental disorders (American Psychiatric Association, 2000). Based on current research and evolving understandings of neurodevelopmental disorders, the American Psychiatric Association (2013) does not currently utilize a separate diagnostic category of Asperger's disorder, which has been subsumed under the current neurodevelopmental diagnosis of ASD.

Despite the diagnostic changes established by the American Psychiatric Association in 2013, Asperger's disorder is currently recognized by the World Health Organization (2014) and remains an important functional clinical diagnosis. As such, a brief overview of Asperger's syndrome is warranted in the context of ASD.

Although Asperger's syndrome is similar in some ways to ASD, there are some important differences between the two clinical syndromes. In general, individuals with Asperger's disorder typically function better than do those with autism. In addition, individuals with Asperger's syndrome generally have normal intelligence and near-normal language development, although there are typically noted deficits in some areas of higher-order language processing and understanding such as pragmatic and contextual language functions (Atwood, 1998; Ghaziuddin, 2005). Unlike the withdrawal from the rest of the world that can be characteristic of individuals with low-functioning autism, children and adults with Asperger's disorder may be more isolated as a result of deficient social skills and narrow interests (Atwood, 1998, 2008). It has been demonstrated that individuals with Asperger's syndrome may have exceptional talents and skills in particular areas, such as music or math (Atwood, 2008).

Symptoms

The symptoms of Asperger's disorder can range from mild to severe, with a common profile (see Table 6.2; Atwood, 1998, 2008; DeOrnellas et al., 2010; Ghaziuddin, 2005).

TABLE 6.2 ASPERGER'S SYNDROME SYMPTOMS

- Problems with social skills: Individuals with Asperger's disorder generally have difficulty interacting with others and can often be awkward in social situations. Many with the disorder have challenges with initiating and maintaining conversations and with developing personal relationships and friendships.

  Individuals with Asperger's syndrome may lack the ability to modulate voice volume to appropriately match situations and surroundings. For example, they may have to be reminded to talk more softly in a classroom or movie theater. Individuals with Asperger's disorder commonly have problems understanding language in context and subsequently can be very literal and ineffective in their use of language in various communication and learning situations.

- Eccentric or repetitive behaviors: Individuals with Asperger's disorder may present with repetitive patterns of odd behaviors and movements, which may be similar to behavioral profiles in some individuals with autism.

- Limited range of interests: It is quite common for individuals with Asperger's disorder to develop intense interest in a particular topic or a few topics that they focus on obsessively and continuously. For instance, a child with the disorder may constantly obsess verbally and otherwise on a topic such as dinosaurs or the weather, and may continuously discuss the preferred subject, even when irrelevant or inappropriate in a given interpersonal interaction.

  Individuals with Asperger's disorder may collect enormous amounts of factual information about their favorite subject and talk incessantly about it. However, the conversation may seem like a random collection of information with no apparent point or conclusion.

- Unusual preoccupations or rituals: An individual with Asperger's disorder may develop and continuously use rituals, such as following a specific sequence of behaviors in daily activities such as eating or getting dressed.
- Coordination problems: It is not unusual for individuals with Asperger's disorder to have gross or fine motor difficulties or delays, which may be observed as awkwardness or clumsiness.
- Difficulties perceiving the perspective of others: Individuals with Asperger's disorder may have difficulties understanding or even being aware of the perspectives, feelings, or experiences of others. Such individuals may consequently have general difficulties in experiencing empathy for others, as a result of cognitive deficits related to the disorder.

Educational Implications

Given many of the crossover symptoms and cognitive and learning problems shared by Asperger's disorder and ASD, many of the educational interventions and accommodations that are helpful to learners with autism will also benefit students with Asperger's syndrome (Atwood, 2008). As previously stated, individuals with Asperger's syndrome commonly have problems with aspects of higher-order language processing, especially involving receptive, expressive, and pragmatic language, and language discourse. Receptive language deficiencies may manifest as problems with figurative and literal language, and even humor and sarcasm. A child with Asperger's disorder may speak quite eloquently and precociously, but may not really understand many of the phrases and grammatical concepts being used (Atwood, 1998, 2008; DeOrnellas et al., 2010; Ghaziuddin, 2005). Discourse involves the understanding and usage of appropriate rules of language and speaking, and in individuals with the disorder, such difficulties may also interfere with learning components of language arts. All of those deficiencies may also contribute to difficulties in interpersonal interactions and general social functioning (Atwood, 1998).

CASE STUDY 6.2: LIAM

Liam is a 12-year-old boy who lives with his biological parents and attends public school in his community, where he is in the sixth grade. He was born full term with no complications, and parent reports indicate no notable early or recent medical concerns for for their son.

Liam's reported developmental history indicated no delays in language development. His parents in fact reported that their son quickly developed a strong vocabulary and was quite articulate and verbally fluent in his preschool years. During his elementary school years, Liam continued to have strong conversation skills, more often with adults, in which he precociously used his extensive vocabulary knowledge. Liam's early and continuing fine-motor and gross-motor development was described as normal, but his parents remarked that he always seemed somewhat uncoordinated, and he always shied away from sport and related physical activities.

By the ages of 4 and 5, his parents began to notice that Liam's patterns of behavioral and social functioning and his general interpersonal and functional communication skills were atypical for children his age. Liam always seemed most comfortable when his days and routines were consistent and highly structured. When he experienced even minimal unexpected changes in plans or routines, he would often become visibly upset and at times subsequently act out behaviorally with oppositional behavior or even tantrums. Liam also reportedly often acted visibly uncomfortable and even emotionally distressed during his preschool years in situations of excessive sound and visual stimulus, such as the shopping mall during the holiday season. Those concerns were also noted more recently when Liam was in elementary school.

By the time he entered elementary school, Liam's difficulties interacting and socializing with his peers became more progressively evident. His teachers noted that, despite his precocious vocabulary and conversation skills, Liam frequently misunderstood interactions and communications with other children. Liam has often been observed to have difficulties following socially accepted rules of conversation, as he typically interrupts others while speaking and frequently appears to be unaware of conversational dynamics.

Liam has been observed over his school years in the context of both peer and teacher-student interactions to misunderstand metaphorical language, usually expressed by adults, such as, "You can throw your coat in that closet." He has exhibited even more difficulty understanding language and visual components of sarcasm. In other words, Liam is very literal and concrete in his thinking, reasoning, and functional usage of language, despite his very good vocabulary knowledge and usage. Liam's parents have long been concerned that their son has great difficulties understanding the perspectives of other children and adults. For instance, when asked how he thinks another individual may feel about a situation, Liam typically answers with honesty only how he obviously feels, and he cannot truly conceptualize another point of view or a different emotional response in others. As a result, Liam's interpersonal skills and capabilities have always been an area of difficulty for him, and those problems have become more significant throughout Liam's later elementary grades.

His parents reported that since his preschool years, Liam has always been obsessively focused on specific topics. As he has become older, that characteristic has intensified. For the past 4 years, Liam has been obsessed with dinosaurs. He collects books and figurines and speaks about dinosaurs constantly. He very often will start speaking about dinosaurs or bring them up in conversations that have nothing to do with them. If he is allowed to do so, Liam will speak about dinosaurs constantly, to the exclusion of appropriate on-topic dialogues with others. All adults who interact with Liam have learned to gently redirect his conversation to more appropriate topics in social and learning situations.

When he was in grade 3, Liam was referred for a special education evaluation by his school system. Due to ongoing classroom performance difficulties, he was falling behind in his academic skills and progress. Despite his obvious strong fundamental reading skills at the word level, Liam was beginning to exhibit academic delays in reading comprehension abilities and written language skills and knowledge. Liam was also beginning, even in grade 3, to present with very noticeable organizational and executive function-related difficulties, which were more evident in school. His parents and most recent teachers expressed concerns that Liam frequently had difficulties following verbal multistep directions, and his teachers have more recently noted patterns of inconsistency in his learning and testing performance. Liam also displayed increasing difficulty remaining attentive and focused at developmentally appropriate levels, especially when he was required to be attentive to academic activities that he did not prefer. These issues prompted Liam's teachers and his parents to consider a primary diagnosis of ADHD.

Liam's evaluation process in grade 3 included a comprehensive battery of assessment procedures that included intellectual, psychological and emotional, neurodevelopmental (learning and memory), and academic achievement testing. The information obtained from his cognitive testing indicated that Liam's overall intellectual abilities were above average for his age, with developmentally very strong overall perceptually based reasoning and processing capabilities. Liam's general language-based learning and processing capacities were inconsistent, based on information from cognitive and comprehensive language evaluation. More specifically, Liam demonstrated unusual strengths in vocabulary knowledge and more fundamental language processes. The assessment data, however, indicated that Liam had developmental language delays in numerous areas of higher-order language concepts and processes, especially in understanding metaphorical language and thinking, multiplicity of word meanings, multiple meanings contained in syntax and grammar structures, and contextual language usage and meanings. Liam's speed and accuracy of applied visual processing and integrated visual-motor processing were noted as significant areas of strength for him. Significant developmental delays were noted regarding his ability to initially learn, process, store, and retrieve information across language and visual modalities. Academic strengths were noted regarding Liam's fundamental reading skills (at the word level) and in regard to his applied math calculation and conceptual math knowledge and skills. Academic delays were evident involving Liam's reading comprehension abilities and in his written language skills, especially involving applied usage of syntax and grammar structure concepts and organizational writing capabilities.

Occupational testing did not provide evidence of any significant visual-perceptual, visual-spatial, or visual-motor developmental deficits. The assessment process also included several parent- and teacher-reported behavioral and emotional rating scales, in addition to a similar scale to investigate a possible diagnosis of Asperger's syndrome. The information obtained from both the parent- and teacher-reported Asperger's syndrome scales indicated a high probability that Liam has that disorder.

Based on the information and findings from this assessment process, Liam was given a primary diagnosis of Asperger's syndrome with a secondary diagnosis of ADHD. The evaluation report raised the possibility that Liam's attentional difficulties in school might be more related to his primary diagnosis of Asperger's syndrome. The professionals working with Liam determined that it was important to focus Liam's concurrent diagnosis of ADHD in addition to his many other concerns, and that those issues needed to be educationally addressed. Liam's clear primary diagnosis of Asperger's syndrome provided a solid framework for the development of comprehensive and educational interventions and supports for him based on best-practice research. His Individualized Educational Plan (IEP) was expanded based on the new diagnostic information and implemented throughout all aspects of his educational programming. Some of the new information included in Liam's IEP, based on his diagnosis of dyspraxia, includes the following.

Liam's daily and weekly routines in school were kept as clear and consistent as possible and appropriate. When routine changes were unavoidable, Liam was provided with additional guidance and supports to help him to better manage more unstructured times and transitions.

All educators working with Liam became more mindful that he had trouble understanding language that is not very literal, but can be more ambiguous and contextually relevant. As such, all of his teachers focused on using very specific instructions and concrete language when communicating with him, while analogies, metaphors, and sarcasm. They were also mindful of being as verbally explicit and direct as possible when communicating with Liam regarding the perspectives and feelings of others.

Liam's educational programming included intensive speech and language services, with a focus on understanding and application of higher-order language concepts. Those teachings were consistently practiced and reinforced across all of Liam's academic activities and educationally related social interactions.

Liam was provided with individual ongoing instruction specifically focused on the development of more effective reading comprehension abilities and skills. Those remedial instructions provided strategies to better enable Liam to monitor his understanding of what he reads and how to extract main ideas in text.

To address his difficulties and delays in written language, it was noted and understood by all educators working with him that Liam's writing difficulties involve all aspects of the writing process that involve higher-order language understanding and organizational writing, including applied knowledge of syntax, grammar, punctuation, and organizational writing procedures. As such, interventions and considerations for Liam's writing deficits were multifaceted and encompassed a range of educational accommodations, modifications, and remediations, which included the following.

To address the complexity of writing, Liam was provided with consistent individualized training focused on developing a systematic process approach to writing. To that end, Liam was taught and allowed ample opportunities to practice how to develop and generate initial drafts of writing based on a primary general outline, He was taught and encouraged to practice and use various techniques to allow him to brainstorm ideas and then systematically organize that written information into outlines and various graphic representations. Liam was progressively taught and allowed to practice a range of sequential and organizational writing strategies that helped him to more effectively break down writing tasks and assignments into organized and manageable steps, and allowed for more systematic ways of developing and utilizing multiple and sequential edits when writing for organization of ideas, content, grammar, syntax, punctuation, and spelling. Consistent feedback was provided to Liam by his teachers on all of those processes throughout his academic day and were consistently reinforced in the contexts of his daily classroom work and his homework.

Liam was also provided with extensive individualized instruction and training in the use of word processing programs, with a specific focus on learning and utilizing various writing tools common in word processing such as "cut and paste" and "spell check" functions.

Liam's educational programming also included weekly participation in a social skills group with a small group of other students with similar difficulties and issues.

Liam's organizational difficulties initially were addressed by the teachers and school environment. Liam benefited from regular daily help with these difficulties. It was helpful for Liam to have someone he could work with at the end of the school day, who consistently checked with him regarding assignments, including making sure Liam knew the steps involved, where to begin, what materials were needed, how much time it should take, and how to assess when each step and final product was completed.

The following accommodations were implemented across all of Liam's educational activities and environments to address his difficulties with attention and focus. In all of his classes, Liam was provided with simple instructions, which his teachers verified that he understood. He had a highly structured learning environment in all of his classes. Information was broken down and presented to Liam through brief, manageable, and meaningful units. When appropriate and possible, all of his educational instructions were utilized using a multisensory approach to learning to enhance, reinforce, and consolidate learning. When appropriate and possible, his instruction utilized a spiral learning approach, in which new learning was based on previously learned material and was periodically reviewed.

As a result of the remedial interventions, instructions, and accommodations in his IEP and the subsequent training and support from all educators working with him, Liam made significant and notable gains in reading comprehension skills and all other academic content areas. His overall daily performance in school was notably better, and his general functioning in class over time progressively improved. Liam was consistently observed to enjoy school more, and his new comfort levels in all of his educational environments in conjunction with specific social skill instructions enhanced his ability to positively connect and interact with peers in and out of the classroom.

Chapter 7

MOTOR DISORDERS

Motor disorders, in the context of neurodevelopmental frameworks, include all integrated and interrelated fine motor, gross motor, and visual-motor skills, which are important across a wide range of learning and educational processes. Various clinical and neurodevelopmental syndromes are encompassed by the general category of motor disorders, which include developmental coordination disorder, dyspraxia, stereotypical movement disorder, tic disorders, and Tourette disorder (American Psychiatric Association, 2013; Ball, 2002; Boon, 2010; Decker & Davis, 2010; Jones, 2005; Kirby & Drew, 2003).

Developmental theorists and related psychological models have provided a foundation of theories and stages of human developmental functions and processes across the life span. Such theories and models include integrated stages of cognitive, motor, and social developmental processes (Farran & Karmil-off-Smith, 2012; Goswami, 2008; Meece & Daniels, 2008; Spreen et al., 1995).

Foundational theories posited by the ground-breaking developmental theorist Jean Piaget outline early stages of such integrated developmental processes (Ginsburg & Opper, 1987; Piaget, 1972). The role of developing neuromotor functions, according to Piaget's theories, are primary during the first two years of life. Piaget posited that during that period of development, which he named the sensorimotor stage, an infant's knowledge of the world is primarily limited to his or her sensory perceptions and motor activities, and developing understanding and learning are strongly related to simple motor responses caused by sensory stimuli that a child utilizes to gain understanding of the environment and the self (Ginsburg & Opper, 1987; Meece & Daniels, 2008; Piaget, 1972).

While neuromotor processes (including developing fine motor and gross motor skills) appear to play a primary role in early childhood development and learning, the developing neuromotor functions and processes continue to be important components of learning and understanding across later developmental stages and indeed across the human life span (Drew & Creek, 2005; Farran & Karmiloff-Smith, 2012; Goswami, 2008; Spreen et al., 1990). While a child may be utilizing integrated visual-spatial and spatial-ordering cognitive constructs while pursuing a puzzle-making task, such a pursuit also typically involves an important degree of neuromotor functions that cooperatively integrate with various other cognitive and motor functions (Ball, 2002; Kurtz, 2007). Consider that many tasks, from producing written language (by hand or computer keyboard) to playing a musical instrument, to performing virtually any athletic endeavor involves a complex integration of neuromotor functions and cognitive processes that also facilitate visual-spatial and spatial ordering constructs, and in some cases (such as in the production of written language) also incorporate higher-order thinking and reasoning capabilities (Feifer & DeFina, 2002; Jongmans, 2005).

DEVELOPMENTAL COORDINATION DISORDER

Developmental coordination disorder has been recognized and clinically described for at least 100 years under various diagnostic categories. The terms used over the past century have included motoric deficiency, minimal brain dysfunction, sensori-integrative dysfunction, perceptuo-motor dysfunction, visuo-motor deficiencies, spatial problems, visuo-motor difficulties, clumsy child syndrome, and developmental dyspraxia (Ball, 2002; Pennington, 2009; Tupper & Sondell, 2004). It may be helpful to understand and remember that all of the terms and diagnostic labels for such problems in children and adults in general refer to movement and related specific aspects of learning (Ball, 2002; Chambers et al., 2005; Drew & Creek, 2005; Kurtz, 2007; Shah & Donald, 1986; Sugden & Shambers, 2005; Walsh et al., 2013).

In addition to understanding developmental coordination disorder as a neurodevelopmental disability characterized by an impairment, immaturity, or disorganization of movement, it is also important to understand that such motor-related disabilities commonly include other learning problems involving language, perceptions, various specific learning disabilities (e.g., in reading, written language, and math), and personality and behavior problems (Ball, 2002; Boon, 2010; Decker & Davis, 2010; Jones, 2005; Kirby & Drew, 2003; Ripley, 2001; Yeo, 2003).

Problems in motor functions and coordination can also be associated with specific neurological disorders such as cerebral palsy, muscular dystrophy, and lesions and tumors in the brain, and in those situations deficits in movement and related functions should be considered within the contexts of those primary medical conditions (Kirby & Drew, 2003; Teeter & Semrud-Clikeman, 2007).

DYSPRAXIA

While the clinical terms and diagnostic labels "developmental coordination disorder" and "dyspraxia" have both been used to describe various motor disorders and related learning problems, differences in motor dysfunctions and deficits have been noted between the two clinical syndromes. These differences have implications for learning. In general, children with developmental coordination disorder can be thought of as having developmental delays and deficits primarily involving motor coordination and execution. Children with developmental dyspraxia can be understood as having problems and developmental delays involving the organization and planning of movement to achieve a predetermined idea or purpose, which may affect the acquisition of new skills and the execution of those already learned. Dyspraxia as a condition, then, can be understood in general as an impairment or developmental delay in the organization of movement.

What Is Praxis?

"Praxis" (which is a linguistic component of the word "dyspraxia") is a Greek word meaning movement (Boon, 2010). We can think of the processes of praxis as a link between our cognitive processes (our brain and thinking functions) and our physical actions and behaviors.

Consider that most of our functioning in the physical world, from the simplest to the most complicated of tasks, requires a complex interaction and subsequent sequential implementation of integrated cognitive and motor functions. Those processes involve ideation (the formation of an idea from a movement that is already learned and internalized), motor planning (planning an action to achieve an idea), and execution (executing a task and sequentially carrying out the ideas and plans necessary for task completion) (Ball, 2002; Boon, 2010; Kirby & Drew, 2003). Another way to think of this is that if an individual wants to formulate ideas and then plan and execute them effectively (from the simple to the most complex), he or she needs to have those combined abilities from previous learned experiences. It is also important to note that processes of praxis are also dependent on innate biological factors unique to each individual, and that such genetic factors occur across all social, ethnic, racial, and cultural boundaries (Gallahue, 1992; Ripley, 2001).

The processes of ideation, motor planning, and execution in the context of praxis are interdependent, and also depend on an ability to accurately recall neurological information obtained from sensory information and experience (Kurtz, 2007). The term "neurological" in this context can be understood as all of the biologically based mental and physical processes that occur in an individual facilitating any mental or physical actions, which are dependent on the availability of the appropriate physiological pathways and connections (Boon, 2010; Drew & Creek, 2005; Kurtz, 2007). Dyspraxia, then, can be understood as a breakdown in the processes of praxis, occurring when sensory information and the motor and mental actions involving ideation, planning, and execution are not biologically coordinated and ultimately do not result in intended physical or mental actions (Kirby & Drew, 2003).

Dyspraxia may affect many areas of development, including intellectual, language, sensory-motor, and even emotional and social. Thus, a diagnosis of dyspraxia in a child or adult may present in varying and even quite different ways among individuals and across different stages of an individual's physical and cognitive development (Ball, 2002; Boon, 2010; Drew & Creek, 2005; Kurtz, 2007).

Boon (2010) describes different types or aspects of dyspraxia that include verbal dyspraxia, sensory integrative dysfunction, and ideational and ideomotor dyspraxia. The term "verbal dyspraxia" is most commonly used when praxis difficulties result in a child having problems and delays in the actual production and formulation of speech sounds and processes. Verbal praxis–related problems may also manifest as difficulties sequencing words in proper order and recalling words accurately when needed in oral language processes (Boon, 2010). "Sensory integrative dysfunction" refers to difficulties organizing information received from various sensory apparatus involving the interaction between internal physical processes and the environment (Ayers, 1972), which can include making sense of physical senses and processes such as sight, hearing, smell, touch, taste, balance, and movement.

Boon (2010) also described a range of difficulties experienced by children with dyspraxia that include developmental deficits and delays in gross and fine motor skills, integrated visual-motor skills and functions, speech and language development and processes, attention and concentration abilities, general learning abilities, and social and emotional development and functioning. Kirby and Drew (2003) also stated that dyspraxia commonly involves other conditions and problems (which can also be described by the more clinical term "comorbidity") that include higher-order language delays and deficits, attention deficit disorder, and specific learning disorders in reading, written language, and mathematics.

CASE STUDY 7.1: EDWARD

Edward is a 9-year-old boy with a history of early developmental delays and academic difficulties since he was in kindergarten. He attends public school in his community, and is in the third grade. Edward's most notable difficulties, from a very early age and throughout elementary school, have involved fine-motor and gross-motor activities and functions, and related problems with coordination and related skills. He commonly has problems with learning activities involving physical handwriting, drawing and paper cutting, and all sports-related activities that involve movement, balance, and running.

In grades 1 and 2, Edward's teachers noted that he appeared to have acquired a solid foundation of cognitive skills related to early reading abilities. More specifically, his applied phonological processing capabilities and related phonics skills seemed developmentally intact, and he appeared to have adequate word automaticity capacities that would support grade equivalent reading fluency abilities. Nevertheless, his teachers reported reading difficulties at the word level, including losing his place, skipping lines, and poor understanding.

Edward has always had difficulties writing letters and words, and academic tasks involving writing continue to be very slow and laborious for him. Even when he is allowed extra time for writing tasks, Edward reportedly has problems lining up words and rows of words on a line, difficulties organizing sentences and paragraphs, and inefficient use of punctuation and grammar rules. In general, when Edward is asked to verbally present a story or information, he usually does so quite well for his age and grade level. When he is required to organize his thoughts and ideas in a written format, however, his writing is developmentally poor.

Edward appears to have a developmentally adequate fund of math calculation skills and applied conceptual math knowledge, but he has always had difficulties performing most math activities and related problem-solving challenges. For instance, his teachers have noted that Edward typically has great difficulty aligning rows of numbers in an equation, and even more difficulty when he attempts to carry over numbers in rows and keep track of accurate sum and minus equations, even though he often can verbalize a conceptual understanding of the math processes that he is employing.

Edward also has difficulty organizing himself, following directions, and maintaining attention. Those issues, along with apparent patterns of hyperactive behavior, have raised concerns that Edward has ADHD. His parents brought those concerns to Edward's pediatrician recently, and Edward was subsequently briefly prescribed a trial medication for attentional regulation, with unsatisfactory results. Most of the educators working with Edward believe that while he may have at least a degree of ADHD, that diagnosis does not explain all of his past and current educational difficulties.

While his academic difficulties have been partially a mystery to his teachers, since grade 1 Edward has had an IEP that provides special educational supports in all of his classes, which are all mainstream classes.

Edward underwent intellectual, cognitive, neurodevelopmental, language, occupational therapy, and academic achievement testing within the past year by his school system. The cognitive testing indicated that Edward's overall intellectual abilities are within an average range for his age. He also presented global language and nonlanguage reasoning and capabilities and general short-term and working memory functions within an average range. Edward's speed and accuracy of applied visual processing and integrated visual-motor processing were noted as significant areas of delay for him. Significant developmental delays were noted regarding Edward's ability to initially learn, process, store, and retrieve information across language and visual modalities. Edward's comprehensive speech and language evaluations indicated that he has developmentally strong language processing and reasoning capacities, which include a good understanding of higher-order language and vocabulary concepts. Edward's academic achievement testing confirmed that his applied phonological processing abilities and related phonics and word decoding skills are developmentally strong, and he has an adequate sight word vocabulary for his grade level. He presented very notable delays, however, involving reading comprehension. Achievement testing also documented very significant delays involving his overall written language skills and knowledge. In addition, despite assessed strong math reasoning abilities, Edward's math calculation skills were very poor.

The occupational therapy testing that Edward underwent provided crucial information related to Edward's problems regarding his academic performance and functioning. That assessment included a developmental history from his parents, in conjunction with standardized testing to assess a broad range of visual-perceptual and visual-motor skills and functions. According to his parents, Edward has learned to perform many age-appropriate skills that involve fine-motor and gross-motor skills, such as tying his shoes and dressing himself, and even simple household chores like sweeping the floor. His parents note, however, that Edward often does not consistently perform many of the tasks he has learned. It is as if he sometimes forgets the sequence of steps to follow. Edward continues to have great difficulty learning age-appropriate physical skills such as riding a bike, and he often appears to be unco-ordinated even when walking and running. Even when he is attempting to be very careful, Edward's general movements often appear clumsy, and his parents describe him as appearing "uncomfortable in his own body" even when he is just sitting. His parents believe that Edward is also quite accident prone for a child his age. Coordination problems were also well documented in school by his teachers and educational specialists in the process of formal occupational therapy.

Standardized test data (using age-based norms) from the occupational therapy assessment presented strong evidence that Edward has dyspraxia, a neurologically based disorder of the processes involving the planning of movement to achieve a predetermined idea or purpose, which may affect the acquisition of new skills and the execution of those already learned. More specifically, Edward's condition involves a disorder of praxis, or the process of ideation (forming an idea of using a known movement to achieve a planned purpose), motor planning (planning the action needed to achieve the idea), and execution (carrying out a planned movement).

Edward's eventual diagnosis of dyspraxia not only helped his teachers and parents better understand his difficulties in school and at home, but provided a clearer framework for the development of comprehensive educational interventions and supports based on best-practice research for the disorder. Edward's IEP was expanded based on the new diagnostic information and implemented throughout all aspects of his educational programming. Some of the new information included in Edward's IEP, based on his diagnosis of dyspraxia, included the following.

The multiple nature of developmental dyspraxia means that educational interventions, academic supports and teaching, and all specific therapies for Edward needed to cover many areas including perceptual motor training, sensory integration therapy, and academic accommodations in reading beyond the word decoding and word identification levels, written language, and math skills.

An occupational therapist began observing how Edward managed with everyday functions both at home and at school. Based on that information, new activities and remedial interventions were included in Edward's educational planning to help him develop and acquire additional skills in activities that were difficult for him. The interventions focused on helping Edward improve body awareness, motor planning skills and strategies, balance skills, fine-motor and gross-motor skills, and functional visual skills, within the context of relevant educational activities. For instance, Edward practiced how to align and work columns of numbers, which relates to fine motor planning skills. Body awareness and balance activities were taught and practiced during Edward's physical education classes. Fine-motor skills were improved through supported activities in art classes.

A more general educational goal was to help Edward develop overall better praxis capabilities. That is, Edward would learn new strategies to help him more effectively and successfully plan, organize, and execute actions across many physical and learning activities.

For Edward, all aspects of reading, writing, and math required a great deal of planning and organization. He was allowed ample opportunities to practice and reinforce those organization and planning skills.

Edward was taught specific strategies to help him more effectively organize and track words in written text. For instance, he used a ruler when reading to help him visually track words, sentences, and paragraphs in text. He learned the same strategies to manipulate columns of numbers during math calculation and problem-solving exercises.

To address his difficulties and delays in written language, his teachers noted that Edward's writing difficulties were not just at the graphomotor or handwriting level but involved all aspects of the writing process (applied knowledge of grammar, syntax, punctuation, and organizational procedures). As such, interventions and considerations for Edward's writing deficits encompassed a range of educational accommodations, modifications, and remediations, which included the following: expected volume of written work, rate of written production, complexity of the writing process, use of various writing tools, and the formatting required.

To address volume of writing, Edward's teachers omitted various grading criteria for written work, such as spelling and good letter formation, and generally allowed for a primary focus on content information and knowledge acquisition.

To address rate of writing involving speed and efficiency on writing tasks, Edward's teachers allowed him extended time whenever possible on tasks involving written language, including homework and longer-term that included any writing. Because of his fine-motor and visual-motor deficits, Edward was provided with individualized computer keyboarding skill training and allowed to type his assignments whenever possible.

To address writing complexity, Edward was provided with consistent individualized training focused on developing a systematic process approach to writing. To that end, Edward was taught how to develop and generate initial drafts based on a primary general outline,

He was taught and encouraged to practice brainstorming ideas and then systematically organizing that written information into outlines and various graphic representations. Edward was progressively taught a range of sequential and organizational writing strategies that helped him to more effectively break down writing tasks and assignments into organized and manageable steps, and allowed for more systematic ways of developing and utilizing multiple and sequential edits when writing for organization of ideas, content, grammar, syntax, punctuation, and spelling. His teachers provided consistent feedback on those processes and consistently reinforced them in the contexts of his daily classroom work and homework.

Edward was also provided with extensive individualized training in the use of word processing programs, with a specific focus on writing tools such as "cut and paste" and "spell check" functions. When he needed to write by hand, Edward was allowed to use writing tools that he was most comfortable with and that best allowed him to write efficiently and effectively, such as erasable pens and pens with large grips.

Finally, whenever possible and appropriate, Edward was offered alternative methods for presenting his classwork and homework and to demonstrate his mastery of knowledge and concepts. For instance, Edward frequently was allowed to take oral tests instead of written tests, and he was encouraged when appropriate to make oral presentations in class.

Given Edward's complex perceptually based developmental delays and related cognitive processing deficits, the following recommendations and accommodations were implemented across all of his educational environments and experiences. All visual materials were simple in format and uncluttered by excessive stimuli. Whenever possible, Edward was assisted in planning and organizing assigned tasks with visual cues (e.g., numbered lines, designated boxes in which to work). When appropriate, teaching techniques began with the identification of individual parts and progressively moved to integrated wholes. Such strategies were also applied to various academic areas, such as math calculation activities and all hands-on types of learning tasks. Whenever possible, all learning modalities were incorporated to stress kinesthetic, visual, and manual manipulation and organizational skills. Edward was given extra opportunities to practice reproducing three-dimensional objects using clay, papier-mâché, or a similar modeling material while looking at a model. He used computer activities and programs designed to develop visual-spatial and visual-motor skills.

Edward's organizational difficulties initially were addressed by the teachers and school environment. Edward benefited from regular daily help from specified individuals at school. At the end of the school day, someone consistently checked with him regarding assignments and making sure Edward knew the steps involved, where to begin, what materials were needed, how much time it should take, and how to assess when each step was completed.

The following accommodations were implemented to address Edward's difficulties with attention and focus. He was provided with a highly structured learning environment in all of his classes. Information was broken down and presented to him through brief, manageable, and meaningful units. He was provided with simple instructions, which teachers verified that he understood. When appropriate and possible, his instruction utilized a spiral learning approach, in which new learning is based on previously learned material and is periodically reviewed. A multisensory approach to learning was used to enhance, reinforce, and consolidate learning.

All of the new remedial interventions, instructions, and accommodations that were added to his IEP and the subsequent training and supports resulted in Edward making significant and notable gains in reading comprehension, overall written language abilities, and general math skills and knowledge. Edward's overall daily performance in school was notably better, and his general functioning in class over time progressively improved. Just as important, Edward appeared to enjoy school more, and his new comfort levels in all of his educational environments seemed to better support not only his academic progress but his ability to more positively connect and interact with peers in and out of the classroom.

STEREOTYPIC MOVEMENT DISORDER

Stereotypic movement disorder is a condition in which an individual engages in repetitive but purposeless movements, which are commonly rhythmic movements of the hands, head, or body. Other common movements related to the disorder include body rocking, head banging, hand shaking and waving, nail-biting, self-hitting, picking at the skin, and mouthing objects (American Psychiatric Association, 2013).

To be considered a disorder, the repetitive movements must continue for at least 4 weeks, and they must interfere with an individual's normal daily functioning (American Psychiatric Association, 2013; Woods & Miltenberger, 2009). Atypical stereotypic movements are commonly also seen in individuals with ASD, tic disorders, obsessive-compulsive disorder, and other neurological and related medical conditions. In those situations deficits in movement and related functions should be considered within the contexts of those primary medical conditions (Minshew & Williams, 2008; Plessen, 2013; Roessner, 2011; Walsh et al., 2013; Shah & Donald, 1986).

TIC DISORDERS

Tics are sudden twitches, movements, or sounds that people do repeatedly and involuntarily (Robertson, 2006; Roessner, 2011; Storch, 2009). Many people experience such spasm-like movements, which often affect the eyelids or face but can also occur anywhere in the body. In most instances, tics and twitches are harmless and temporary, but in some cases such movements may be caused by a tic disorder.

Two types of tics are recognized, which in general are motor tics and vocal tics (American Psychiatric Association, 2013). In episodes of motor and vocal tics, both occur suddenly during what is otherwise normal behavior. Tics are also often repetitive, with numerous successive occurrences of the same action. For instance, someone with a tic might blink his eyes multiple times or twitch her nose repeatedly. Motor tics can be classified as either simple or complex. Simple motor tics may include movements such as eye blinking, head jerking, or shoulder shrugging. Complex motor tics consist of a series of movements performed in the same order. For instance, a person might reach out and touch something repeatedly, or may tap one foot and then the other in a repeating pattern (Freeman & Soltanifar, 2010; Plessen, 2013).

The American Psychiatric Association (2013) divides the neurodevelopmental diagnosis of tic disorders into four diagnostic categories: (1) Tourette disorder, (2) persistent (chronic) motor or vocal tic disorder, (3) provisional tic disorder, and (4) other specified and unspecified tic disorders. The tic disorders differ from each other in terms of the type of tic present (motor or vocal, or a combination of both) and how long the symptoms have lasted. For instance, individuals with Tourette syndrome have both motor *and* vocal tics, and have had tic symptoms for at least one year. Individuals with persistent (chronic) motor or vocal tic disorder have either motor *or* vocal tics, and have had tic symptoms for at least one year. Individuals with provisional tic disorder can have motor or vocal tics, or both, but have had their symptoms less than one year. The following brief overview of three clinical subcategories of tic disorder will aid in the clarification of the diagnostic profile of each disorder.

Tourette Syndrome

Tourette syndrome is a neurological and neurodevelopmental disorder that becomes evident in early childhood or adolescence. The first symptoms usually are involuntary movements (tics) of the face, arms, legs, or trunk of the body.

The involuntary tics of Tourette syndrome may also involve complex body movements, such as kicking and stamping. Other symptoms can also occur, such as touching, repetitive thoughts and movements, and compulsive thoughts and actions. The symptoms of Tourette syndrome typically vary from person to person, and range from very mild to severe, with the majority of cases falling into the mild category (American Psychiatric Association, 2013; Cavanna & Seri, 2013).

Vocal tics also occur with Tourette syndrome, and such actions can include involuntary grunting, throat clearing, shouting, and barking (Cavanna & Seri, 2013; Robertson, 2006). Vocal tics may also be expressed as involuntary use of obscene words or socially inappropriate words and phrases (known as coprolalia) or gestures (known as copropraxia), although those symptoms and behaviors are rather uncommon in Tourette syndrome (National Tourette Syndrome Association, 2014).

It is not unusual for other clinical conditions to co-occur with Tourette syndrome, most commonly ADHD and obsessive-compulsive disorder (Lebowitz, 2012; Plessen, 2013; Robertson, 2006; Storch, 2009).

The National Tourette Syndrome Association (2014) outlines the following clinical guidelines for recognizing the presence of Tourette disorder, based on current diagnostic criteria established by the American Psychiatric Association (2013):

For a person to be diagnosed with Tourette syndrome, he or she must have both multiple motor tics (for example, eye blinking or shoulder shrugging) and vocal tics (for example, repetitive throat clearing, or involuntarily yelling out a word or phrase), although they might not always happen at the same time.

For a person to be diagnosed with Tourette syndrome, he or she must have had tics for at least a year. It is of note that the tics can occur many times a day (usually in bouts) nearly every day, or off and on.

For a person to be diagnosed with Tourette syndrome, he or she must have tics that begin before he or she is 18 years of age.

For a person to be diagnosed with Tourette syndrome, he or she must have symptoms that are not due to taking medicine or other drugs, and not a result of having another medical condition such as a seizure disorder or another neurological or medical condition.

Persistent (Chronic) Motor or Vocal Tic Disorder

Individuals with persistent (chronic) motor or vocal tic disorder have tic symptoms and behaviors that have been observably present for at least one year (American Psychiatric Association, 2013). This neurodevelopmental condition, while similar to Tourette syndrome, is diagnosed when an individual has observable patterns of either motor *or* vocal tics but not both (individuals with Tourette syndrome have both types of tics). As in Tourette syndrome, a diagnosis of persistent (chronic) motor or vocal tic disorder also involves onset before the age of 18. The diagnosis also must rule out a diagnosis of Tourette syndrome, and must also not be due to taking medicine or other drugs, and not a result of having another medical condition such as a seizure disorder (American Psychiatric Association, 2013; Roessner, 2011).

Provisional Tic Disorder

Individuals with provisional tic disorder can have either motor or vocal tics, or both types of tics, but to meet this diagnosis the observable symptoms must not be present for longer than 12 months in a row. As in persistent (chronic) motor or vocal tic disorder, a confirming diagnosis of provisional tic disorder also includes ruling out a diagnosis of Tourette syndrome and persistent (chronic) motor or vocal tic disorder, and must also not be due to taking medicine or other drugs, and not a result of having another medical condition such as a seizure disorder (American Psychiatric Association, 2013; Robertson, 2006).

Chapter 8

NEURODEVELOPMENTAL DISORDERS AND SPECIFIC LEARNING DISABILITIES

The term "learning disability" can be confusing and even anxiety provoking for parents, and misunderstood among educators and professionals across various clinical and medical disciplines. In addition, learning disabilities can be defined and understood differently in different countries, and even within various regions of the United States (Kozey & Seigel, 2008; Learning Disabilities Association of America, 2014; Learning Disabilities Association of Canada, 2014; National Center for Learning Disabilities, 2014; Vargo & Young, 2011a, 2011b).

"Learning disabilities" is actually a general term that describes specific kinds of learning problems. Such a problem, to be considered a type of learning disability, must be primarily related to an individual's innate cognitive abilities and functions, and must not be primarily due to environmental factors (Council for Exceptional Children, 2014; Vargo & Young, 2011b). In other words, an individual with actual learning disabilities is either born with those issues or acquires them through events such as a brain injury. Researchers think that learning disabilities are caused by differences in how a person's brain works and how the brain processes information. Individuals with learning disabilities, in fact, usually have average or above average intelligence, but they process information differently from more typical learners their age (Berninger & Richards, 2002; Fletcher et al., 2007; Pennington, 2009; Yeates et al., 2010). Since the underlying etiologies of learning disabilities are primarily neurological in origin, a learning disability can also be understood as a neurodevelopmental disorder (American Psychiatric Association, 2013).

According to the U.S. National Joint Committee on Learning Disabilities, the term "learning disabilities" refers to a heterogeneous group of disorders manifested by significant difficulties in the acquisition and use of listening, speaking, reading, writing, reasoning, or mathematical abilities. These disorders are intrinsic to the individual, presumed to be due to central nervous system dysfunction, and may occur across the life span. Problems in self-regulatory behaviors, social perception, and social interaction may exist with learning disabilities but do not by themselves constitute a learning disability. Although learning disabilities may occur concomitantly with other handicapping conditions (for example, sensory impairment, mental retardation, serious emotional disturbance) or with extrinsic influences (such as cultural differences, insufficient or inappropriate instruction), they are not the result of those conditions or influences (National Joint Committee on Learning Disabilities, 1988).

Learning disabilities are more common than many people may realize. For instance, it has been documented that as many as one out of every five people in the United States has a recognized form of a learning disability. Consequently, almost 3 million children in the United States (ages 6 through 21) have some form of a learning disability and receive special education in school (Vargo & Young, 2011b). According to the American Psychiatric Association (2013), the prevalence of specific learning disabilities in school-age children across different languages and cultures (across academic domains involving reading, written language, and math) is approximately 5–15%.

DEFINITIONS OF LEARNING DISABILITIES

The Individuals With Disabilities Education Act (IDEA), the U.S. federal special education law (McIntosh & Decker, 2005), defines learning disabilities as follows:

"Specific Learning Disability" means a disorder in one or more of the basic psychological processes involved in understanding or in using language, spoken or written, which may manifest itself in an imperfect ability to listen, think, speak, read, write, spell, or to do mathematical calculations. The term *includes* such conditions as perceptual handicaps, brain injury, minimal brain dysfunction, dyslexia, and developmental aphasia. The term *does not include* children who have learning problems which are primarily the result of visual, hearing, or motor handicaps, of mental retardation, of emotional disturbance, or of environmental, cultural or economic disadvantage.

Children who meet the following criteria are included in the definition of learning disabilities: 1) children who have average to above average intellectual abilities, yet 2) are failing, struggling with, or experiencing significant difficulties in learning one subject or a number of subjects despite exposure to a "normal" teaching environment, and (3) whose learning problems are not secondary to one or more of the exclusions listed in the federal law above (visual, hearing, motor handicaps, mental retardation, emotional disturbance, environmental, cultural or economic disadvantage).

The Learning Disabilities Association of Canada (2014), in January 2002, posited the following definition that frames learning disability diagnosis and educational policies in that country:

Learning Disabilities refer to a number of disorders which may affect the acquisition, organization, retention, understanding or use of verbal or nonverbal information. These disorders affect learning in individuals who otherwise demonstrate at least average abilities essential for thinking and/or reasoning. As such, learning disabilities are distinct from global intellectual deficiency.

Learning disabilities result from impairments in one or more processes related to perceiving, thinking, remembering or learning. These include, but are not limited to: language processing; phonological processing; visual spatial processing; processing speed; memory and attention; and executive functions (e.g. planning and decision-making).

Learning disabilities range in severity and may interfere with the acquisition and use of one or more of the following:

oral language (e.g. listening, speaking, understanding);
reading (e.g. decoding, phonetic knowledge, word recognition, comprehension);
written language (e.g. spelling and written expression);
and mathematics (e.g. computation, problem solving).

Learning disabilities may also involve difficulties with organizational skills, social perception, social interaction and perspective taking.

Other countries also use differing terms to describe these conditions. For example, in the United States and Canada the term "intellectual disability" is used for what is described as a "learning disability" in the United Kingdom. Conditions such as dyslexia (disorders of reading) and disorders of written language and mathematics are recognized by U.K. learning disability organizations and the British Psychological Society (Foundation for People With Learning Disabilities, 2014; Professional Affairs Board of the British Psychological Society, 2000; United Kingdom Department of Health, 2014).

Whatever geographical region you live in and whatever educational systems you are dealing with, there are some fundamental concepts that are commonly accepted involving the understanding of learning. For instance, it is accepted across many international educational systems that individuals with learning disabilities have at least average-range general intelligence, with specific areas of learning problems that can cause trouble in learning and using certain academic and education-related skills (American Speech-Language-Hearing Association, 1991; Council for Exceptional Children, 2014; Foundation for People With Learning Disabilities, 2014; National Center for Learning Disabilities, 2014; World Health Organization, 2014). The educational skill sets most often affected by specific learning disabilities, according to the general consensus reflected by the above national and world organizations, include the following educational and cognitive areas:

- Reading fluency skills
- Reading comprehension
- Written language
- Mathematics calculation
- Mathematics problem solving
- Listening (listening comprehension)
- Speaking (oral expression)
- Reasoning
- Learning and memory

SIGNS OF LEARNING DISABILITIES

Parents and teachers commonly wonder and ask how they can know whether their child or student has a learning disability. While there is no single sign that shows a person has a learning disability, educational and clinical professionals look for a noticeable difference between how well a child does in school and how well he or she could do, given his or her assessed intelligence or ability (Vargo & Young, 2011a). There are many signs that may indicate that a child has a learning disability, and many of those signs become apparent in elementary school, when a child is increasingly required to demonstrate learning skills and knowledge (Vargo & Young, 2011b). If a child is showing a number of such specific problems, then parents and teachers should consider the possibility that the child has a learning disability.

The following is a list of questions (most here specific to elementary grades, but many applicable for adolescents and adults) that parents can ask a teacher to determine the likelihood that their child may have a learning disability:

- Does my child have trouble learning the alphabet, rhyming words, or connecting letters to their sounds?
- Does my child have difficulties for his or her age sounding out and decoding words and letter combinations?
- Does my child have trouble remembering the sounds that letters make or hearing slight differences between words?
- Does my child often mispronounce words or use a wrong word that sounds similar?
- Does my child make many mistakes when reading aloud, and does he or she repeat and pause often when reading orally?
- Is my child having difficulty understanding what he or she reads?
- Is my child having difficulty with spelling?
- Does my child have very poor handwriting, or does he or she hold a pencil awkwardly for his or her age?
- Is my child having difficulties understanding and using fundamental rules of grammar, syntax, and punctuation when writing?
- Is my child showing great difficulty expressing ideas in writing?

- Is my child having difficulties with organizing his or her thoughts when attempting to write?
- Does my child appear to have difficulties following verbal directions?
- Does my child appear to have difficulties making himself or herself understood by using language; for instance, is he or she able to verbalize feelings, frustrations, and so on at a developmentally appropriate level?
- Does my child appear to have a limited developing vocabulary for his or her age?
- Does my child appear to have trouble organizing what he or she wants to say at a developmentally appropriate level?
- Does my child often appear unable to think of the word he or she needs when speaking or writing?
- Does my child appear to have trouble understanding jokes, comic strips, stories, and sarcasm at a developmentally appropriate level?
- Is my child often unable to retell a story in order and in the appropriate sequence initially presented?
- Is my child showing difficulties following the social rules of conversation—for instance, appropriately taking turns when conversing with another, standing at an appropriate distance from a listener, and so on?
- Is my child having difficulties memorizing and using math facts at appropriate grade levels, for instance, memorizing the times tables, and so on?
- Is my child having difficulty understanding and applying grade-appropriate mathematical concepts and ideas?
- Does my child appear to be having difficulties knowing where to begin a task and then following through with the organization and process of completing that task?
- Is my child having difficulty in class remaining focused and attentive at a developmentally appropriate level?

A teacher who observes a child over time in a classroom setting can provide parents with valuable information about how he or she is able to learn and function in school in all of the ways that he or she should be able to for his or her age and grade level. If a teacher and parents feel that a child has apparent problems learning to read, write, listen, speak, or do math, then it is appropriate to further investigate those concerns. Such investigations may appropriately include a comprehensive evaluation by appropriate professionals, such as a neuropsychologist, school psychologist, and special education specialist to clarify specific learning problems and also to rule out any other issues that may be affecting a student's educational progress and functioning.

Chapter 9

SPECIFIC LEARNING DISORDERS IN READING

Writing symbols have been used to represent human speech and ideas for more than 5,000 years. Reading as a structured system has only existed for a few thousand years (Berninger & Wolf, 2009; Wolf, 2007). Reading in fact is an invention of humans, as we apparently are not designed by evolutionary processes to be readers (Wolf, 2007). Nevertheless, reading remains one of the single most important inventions of our species, which expanded our abilities cognitively, academically, technologically, and historically (Wolf, 2007). Across all languages and cultures, reading processes involve a complex interaction of cognitive and physiological processes that include many facets of language and memory functions (Benasich & Fitch, 2012; Feifer, 2010; Feifer & DeFina, 2000; Henderson, 2012; Vargo, 2007). Reading processes at many levels facilitate word recognition and understanding for multiple levels of text comprehension (Berninger & Richards, 2002; Berninger & Wolf, 2009).

Disorders of reading, when not caused primarily by environmental factors such as limited opportunities to learn and develop age-appropriate academic skills, are neurologically based (Hynd & Cohen, 1983; Vargo, 2007; Vargo et al., 2008). Hence, a reading disability, as well as the alternate diagnostic framework of developmental dyslexia, can also be understood as a neurodevelopmental disorder (American Psychiatric Association, 2013).

The term "dyslexia," while commonly recognized and frequently used by educators and parents, is ambiguous and often misused and misunderstood (Vargo et al., 2004). Some parents, teachers, and even physicians may believe that dyslexia only involves reversed letters or reading backward. Such misunderstandings can then lead to confusion regarding diagnosis of the disorder, and to subsequent problems regarding appropriate remedial interventions and educational accommodations. Issues surrounding diagnostic and remedial factors are also compounded by the recognized heterogeneity and complexity of reading disorders (Hynd & Cohen, 1983; Shaywitz, 2003).

It is also currently understood that reading disabilities can be conceptualized as a syndrome that follows a dimensional model. That is, disorders of reading typically occur on a continuum, with a range of reading difficulties that vary in degree as well as in nature. Nevertheless, reading disabilities are often diagnosed by educational systems within the context of a categorical model, which posits that dyslexia is a discrete disorder that one either has or does not have, and that can be accurately identified by utilizing arbitrarily established criteria (Shaywitz, 2003).

The clinical investigation of possible reading-disordered individuals (as well as individuals with other types of learning disabilities) utilizing the context of a rigid (and often arbitrary) categorical model can often result in inaccurate and incomplete diagnoses of reading deficiencies and often inappropriate remedial interventions for children and adults who do indeed have significant innate reading problems (Spafford & Grosser, 1996; Vargo, 2007).

Since the processes of reading are complex and multifaceted, it follows that developmental delays and deficits in cognitive functions that support reading processes can result in reading delays or disabilities of varying degrees and natures (Benasich, 2012; Benasich & Fitch, 2012; Feifer, 2010; Feifer & DeFina, 2000; Henderson, 2012; Shaywitz, 2003; Vargo, 2007). The following sections outline the primary functions that support reading processes and that can contribute to reading delays and deficits.

READING AND PHONOLOGICAL PROCESSING

Phonological processing refers to an individual's overall innate ability to hear, discriminate, recognize, and understand the various sound components in language (Kamhi & Catts, 1989; Vargo et al., 1995, 2004). Phonological awareness, the ability to hear and understand the sound-symbol correspondences of the printed page, is a critical component of early reading development (Rayner & Pollatsek, 1989). Phonological awareness is also referred to as linguistic or phonemic awareness. Phonological awareness is considered an important predictor of future reading abilities and reading problems (Vargo, 1992, 2007; Wagner et al., 1999). Young students who are dyslexic, or at the very least have beginning reading problems, frequently experience difficulty in phonological awareness and processing abilities in general (Wagner et al., 1999).

The term "phonics" is often confused with phonological processing and phonemic awareness. Phonics, however, refers to a learned set of skills involving a reader's ability to sound out, read, and spell according to a specific set of rules (Spafford & Grosser, 1996). Another way to understand the differences between those terms is to think of phonological processing abilities as innate capacities that an individual normally has a natural ability to learn and develop, while phonics is reading-related skills that involve phonemic awareness, but that have to be learned and practiced. It should be obvious that a young reader's ability to effectively develop age-appropriate phonics skills can be compromised by a developmental deficit in any areas of phonological processing. The importance of assessing the range of possible phonologically based difficulties and deficiencies in early (and older) struggling readers should also be apparent.

A brief overview of the various components of phonological processing and awareness, and the linguistic processes involved, may help to facilitate a broader understanding of the reading process and phonologically based reading problems. Such an overview can also provide a foundation for a better understanding of often-used terminologies, effective assessment techniques, and remedial interventions for reading deficiencies.

Phonemes and Phonological Awareness

The most fundamental components of language itself are sounds within words, called phonemes. Phonemes represent differences in speech sounds that reflect differences in meaning. For instance, individuals attending to everyday conversations hear and understand different phonemes in the speech stream, and those perceived phonemes facilitate understanding from verbal information. The English language contains around 44 phonemes.

Speech itself is made up of strings of "phones," or basic sounds of a language. Phones are actually sets of speech sounds that are found in all languages (Wagner et al., 1999). An individual phone represents a specific combination of articulatory gestures in the speech process, for instance, tongue placement during speech, vocal cord vibrations, and mouth position.

Words are combinations of these component sounds that are bound and blended together in a variety of ways. In essence, phonemes are the building blocks of words. Some examples of phonemes in the English language are as follows:

Language Sound	Letter	Word Example
Short vowel	e	leg
Long vowel	a	pay
Consonant	n	new
Consonant blend	scr	scratch
Vowel digraph	ea	teach

Beginning readers vary widely in their ability to hear and understand the subtle differences between phonemes (Levine, 2002; Spafford & Grosser, 1996). A child's ability to distinguish and sort out the sound components in words is related to his or her phonological awareness process. The term "phonemic awareness" is often used to describe a young reader's ability to specifically process the phonemic components in a word (Levine, 2002). Children who are at a developmentally appropriate level of phonemic awareness at the early stages of reading should be developing a solid ability to divide a word into its most fundamental language sounds and then reblend those sounds to create a different word.

The process of breaking apart and then reorganizing the sound components in words is commonly referred to as word segmentation and reblending. Young readers need to have a solid foundation of word segmentation and reblending abilities to facilitate word decoding skills. Word decoding refers to the ability to apply phonological capabilities to sound out and identify familiar and unfamiliar words.

Phonological Memory and the Role of Memory Functions

Another important component of phonological processing is phonological memory. Phonological memory refers to a reader's ability to code phonological information for temporary storage in working or short-term memory (Vargo, 1992). An example is the temporary remembering of a phone number for a minute until one can actually dial it. Most individuals will (without really thinking about it) continue to repeat the series of numbers until they can be dialed. The utilization of that strategy allows for the employment of phonological memory to facilitate a brief and temporary remembering of a phone number.

Correlating research documents the importance of working memory functions to reading abilities (Kamhi & Catts, 1989; Swanson, Cochran, & Eivers, 1990; Torgeson, 1988; Torgeson & Houck, 1990; Vargo, 1992; Vargo et al., 1995). For instance, findings have shown that when verbal and verbally recoded information is stored in working memory, the stimuli are encoded according to their phonological features (Brady et al., 1983; Torgeson, 1988).

Overall, research has quite impressively shown that many reading-disabled individuals are deficient in the ability to code phonological information in working memory, and that these difficulties may be related to problems in the retrieval of speech sound codes in long-term memory (Kamhi & Catts; 1989; Vargo, 1992; Vargo et al., 1995).

The part of memory that is most involved in the storage of phonological information is most commonly called the phonological loop. This loop allows for a brief storage of auditory information, and it consists of two components working together (Wagner et al., 1999). The first component is the phonological store, which can be likened to a tape-recorded loop that holds 2 seconds of auditory information. The second component is an articulatory control process. One function of this component is to refresh information that is already in the loop so that such information can be stored for longer than 2 seconds.

Phonological memory difficulties alone in developing readers do not appear to impair either reading or listening to a significant extent, providing the words involved are already in the individual's vocabulary. It is important to note, however, that phonological memory impairments can interfere with the ability to learn new written and spoken vocabulary. Deficiencies in phonological memory have also repeatedly been shown to impair development of written and spoken vocabularies in young children (Wagner et al., 1999).

IMPLICATIONS FOR REMEDIAL INTERVENTIONS FOR PHONOLOGICAL PROBLEMS

An important reason for assessing phonological awareness in developing readers suspected of phonological processing delays is that many reading-delayed children have shown improved reading performance after being given remedial interventions that specifically focused on phonological awareness (Wagner et al., 1999). It has been repeatedly shown that remedial reading programs that focus specifically on instructions in phonological awareness and word decoding skills are more successful in improving the reading abilities of children who are weak in such skills, when compared to interventions that do not emphasize phonological awareness (Wagner et al., 1999).

A number of established remedial reading programs focus on the development of phonological awareness and related phonics skills, and special education departments in most school systems will use standard structured reading programs when a student is determined to need help in phonological processing and phonics development. If a parent has questions or concerns regarding the remedial reading programs that a school system uses, the following guide may be helpful.

In a structured remedial program that focuses on instructions in phonological awareness and word decoding skills, reading skills should be explicitly taught using a structured, developmentally progressive system. There are a variety of such linguistic approaches to reading.

Phonological analysis should be explicitly taught, demonstrating how words can be broken down into sounds. In some such programs, for instance, playing with rhymes and multi-sensory representations of sounds through visualizing and tapping them out can promote phonological awareness.

Students appear to learn better when decoding skills are taught using larger chunks, such as word families, where patterns can be emphasized and fewer demands placed on memory.

Reading decoding and word attack strategies need to become automatic. Guessing at words should be discouraged.

Spelling should be taught in conjunction with the reading instruction program, using the same patterns or words utilized in reading.

When a student with significant phonological processing delays is learning within the context of a remedial program, the greatest success occurs when such instructions are given by a qualified, experienced reading specialist, on an individual basis or in a small (two or three individuals) group, and conducted on a daily basis.

CASE STUDY 9.1: EMILY

Emily is an 8-year-old student at the end of the second grade in public school, who was referred for an educational evaluation because of concerns regarding her reading progress and development. According to her current classroom teacher, Emily began the second grade with developmentally weak decoding and phonics skills. She presented clear difficulties hearing the sounds of letters and letter blends. Based on a standard assessment at the beginning of grade 2 utilized by her school system, Emily's beginning phonics skills (her ability to decode and sound out unfamiliar words) were at approximately a beginning first grade level. Emily did appear at the beginning of the second grade to be developing an adequate sight word vocabulary. Her reading skills could seem developmentally sound when she was asked to read high-frequency words common to her grade level. However, when she was presented with less familiar words that were not in her acquired sight word vocabulary, her ability to decode and read those words was clearly delayed for her age.

During her second grade year, her teacher noted that Emily continued to increase her sight word vocabulary, but her decoding skills were showing no improvement. As a result, Emily participated in a computer-based instructional reading program twice a week for 30-minute sessions. Her reading progress was tracked on a weekly basis, and over time it was determined that Emily's reading pattern of good sight word recognition but poor word decoding skills was continuing, despite the additional instruction.

Emily's evaluation process included a comprehensive battery of assessment procedures that included intellectual and cognitive, language, occupational therapy, and academic achievement testing. The cognitive testing indicated that Emily's overall intellectual abilities were within an average range for her age, with developmentally strong overall perceptually based reasoning and processing capabilities. She also had strong visual-speed, visual-scanning, and integrated visual-motor functions, and developmentally adequate learning capacities involving short-term memory and working memory processes. Occupational testing also did not provide evidence of any significant visual-perceptual, visual-spatial, or visual-motor developmental deficits.

Emily's ability to automatically retrieve visual information, a cognitive skill set related to word automaticity capabilities, was within a typical range of development. Her general language-based learning and processing capacities were also developmentally strong. More comprehensive language testing indicated that Emily also had developmentally good receptive and expressive language capabilities.

Academic achievement testing indicated that Emily had an adequate fund of sight-word knowledge for her age, reasonably good beginning overall writing skills and knowledge, and strong math calculation skills and applied math reasoning and knowledge. She presented clear academic delays regarding word decoding, spelling, and reading comprehension.

The assessment data provided strong and consistent evidence that Emily had neurodevelopmental language based-delays involving overall phonological processing abilities, including phonological awareness and memory capabilities. The assessment data helped to identify Emily as a student with a reading disability caused by neurodevelopmental delays in phonological processing abilities and related primary language functions. Emily's word decoding problems, also known as developmental dyslexia, resulted from her delayed ability to hear, understand, and distinguish letter sounds and blends and connect those sounds with visual representations of letters and words.

Based on the assessment process, an IEP was developed for Emily and implemented throughout all aspects of her educational programming, including the following modifications. Reading decoding skills were explicitly taught using a structured, developmentally progressive system. She progressively developed those abilities more effectively when decoding skills were taught to her using larger word and letter combination components such as word families, where patterns can be emphasized and fewer demands placed on memory functions.

Phonological analysis strategies and understandings were explicitly taught to Emily on a daily basis by a qualified reading specialist, individually or in a small group. That instruction involved learning and practicing how to break words down into sounds, and playing with rhymes and multisensory representations of sounds (such as tapping out sound components with the fingers). Emily's spelling instruction was consistently taught in conjunction with her reading instruction program, using the same patterns or words utilized in reading and reading analysis.

The remedial interventions, instruction, and accommodation that were included in her IEP and the subsequent training and support resulted in significant and notable gains in Emily's phonological processing abilities and her related word decoding and general phonics skills. Those academic gains also improved her reading comprehension abilities, spelling skills, and overall written language knowledge and abilities.

READING AND WORD AUTOMATICITY

Research has also discovered compelling and converging evidence that there are primary contributing cognitive factors in addition to phonological processing-related functions that compromise the reading process in some individuals. More specifically, many significantly impaired readers have naming-speed deficits—that is, developmental deficiencies involving the rapid or automatic retrieval of visual information (Manis, Doi, & Bhada, 2000; Wolf & Bowers, 1999; Wolf, Bowers, & Biddle, 2000; Wiig, Zureich, & Chan, 2000).

Word Identification in the Reading Process

An accomplished (adult) reader who picks up the morning newspaper obviously does not sound out each word as it is encountered. To do so would be extremely tedious and slow, and would severely encumber the overall reading process (Rayner & Pollatsek, 1989; Spafford & Grosser, 1996). In reality, an accomplished reader will sequentially scan each word and automatically and instantaneously recognize (and thus read) that word. That process, commonly referred to as word automaticity, is a reader's ability to read fluently. Of course, when an unfamiliar word is encountered, fluent readers may apply phonics skills to decode that word. Repetition of a new word, initially decoded, through repeated reading exposures will eventually encode, or permanently store, the word in an individual's long-term memory (Ashcraft, 1989; Cohen et al., 1986; Matlin, 1989; Schank, 1982; Wagner et al., 1999).

Once a word (in the form of its visual features) is permanently stored, the act of automatically identifying (reading) that word is actually a process of the automatic retrieval of the previously stored visual code of that word (Brady et al., 1983; Schank, 1982; Wiig et al., 2000; Wolf et al., 2000). Despite the notion that it may be a rather simple process, word automaticity actually involves a very complex interaction of cognitive functions and physiological processes (Rayner & Pollatsek, 1989; Schank, 1982; Spafford & Grosser, 1996).

Rapid Naming and Word Retrieval

A large body of scientific evidence, encompassing the past three decades, demonstrates that a majority of children and adults with reading disabilities have difficulties with cognitive tasks recognized collectively as rapid naming tasks (Manis et al., 2000; Wiig et al., 2000; Wolf et al., 2000). The tasks and processes involved in rapid naming procedures include the visual recognition of letters, numbers, colors, and simple objects.

Early scientific investigations of rapid naming processes were conducted in the 1960s by neuroscientist Norman Geschwind. In 1965, Geschwind proposed and then demonstrated that the cognitive components involved in the process of naming colors (attaching a verbal label to an abstract stimulus) were similar to the underlying cognitive components that facilitated some aspects of the reading process at the word level. Hence, observable developmental delays in various rapid naming tasks could be predictive of early reading performance and difficulties. Building on Geschwind's work, Denckla (1972) and Denckla and Rudel (1974) demonstrated that the speed of name retrieval of stimuli, and not necessarily the accuracy of such information recall, differentiated dyslexic (reading-disabled) readers from nondisabled readers.

Differences in naming speed capabilities between dyslexic and developmentally typical readers have also been demonstrated, through extensive international research, across many languages (Wolf et al., 2000). Those findings suggest, among other indications, that the frequent irregularity of the English language (that is, words do not always directly sound like they are spelled according to generally established phonics rules) does not necessarily account for naming speed deficiencies of readers of English (Wolf et al., 2000).

Rapid naming requires speed and processing of visual (orthographic) as well as verbal (phonological) information (Wagner et al., 1999). In fact, research has also posited that the automatic retrieval of phonological information and codes (involving individual phonemes, word segments, and entire words) may facilitate the interactive processes of phonological processing and word decoding (Manis et al., 2000; Vargo et al., 2004; Wagner et al., 1999; Wolf, 1991).

OTHER CONTRIBUTING FACTORS IN READING DYSFLUENCY

Research has presented a range of other cognitive factors that can contribute to dysfluent reading (Adams, 1990; Rayner & Pollatsek, 1989; Spafford & Grosser, 1996; Vargo, 1992; Vargo et al., 1995; Wolf & Katzir-Cohen, 2001; Wolf et al., 2000). Some identified factors from those studies include the following:

- Poor integration of phonological, visuospatial, and working memory functions

- Failure to make higher-order semantic and phonological connections between words, meanings, and ideas
- A breakdown in the processing of syntactic information in written text
- Slow retrieval of names, meaning, or both

READING FLUENCY AND COMPREHENSION

Numerous studies and publications document the relationship between dysfluent reading and impaired reading comprehension (Kamhi & Catts, 1989; Rayner & Pollatsek, 1989; Spafford & Grosser, 1996; Vargo et al., 2004). Reading comprehension is highly dependent on the effective integration of fundamental reading processes at the word level (phonological processing and word decoding skills and word automaticity capacities), and higher-order language capacities that involve the simultaneous processing of syntactic, semantic, and schematic information (Rayner & Pollatsek, 1989; Kamhi & Catts, 1989). A breakdown in the integration of any of those cognitive and language processes will compromise an individual's ability to ultimately successfully process text for meaning and comprehension.

Most commonly, readers who are developmentally struggling with reading words (that is, readers with poor decoding and/or word automaticity skills) are utilizing most of their cognitive capacities to read the words, with little or no mental energy remaining to facilitate and integrate the meanings contained in the words and sentences.

Remedial Interventions for Reading Dysfluency

It has been shown that interventions (especially with early and prereaders) that target specific cognitive functions that facilitate automaticity have been successful in improving the fluency rates, and ultimately the reading process, in children (Hale & Fiorello, 2004; Spafford & Grosser, 1996; Torgeson, Rashotte, &

Alexander, 2001). Some of the most important principles recognized in reading fluency instruction (and emphasized by Torgeson et al.) include anticipatory facilitation, repetition, practice, and outside reading. Of those four general areas, the most established and widely used method to increase reading fluency is the application of repetition through repeated reading techniques (Myer & Felton, 1999). Repeated reading involves both straightforward practice and concurrent instructional support and techniques in which a child repeatedly reads letters, words, phrases, or passages a specific number of times (or until a predetermined level of fluency is reached). According to a report by the National Reading Panel (2000), the repeated reading technique was found to be the only method that yielded consistent and positive effectiveness in increasing reading fluency.

Research has prompted some theorists to present a model of reading fluency as a developmental process that initially precedes and then facilitates the reading process. In that framework, fluency is not regarded as simply an outcome of reading, but rather as a developmental continuum of processes that need to be addressed (in conjunction with early phonemic awareness) before actual reading even begins (Kame'enui, Simmons, Good, & Harn, 2001). The developmental continuum model of reading fluency that begins before the actual reading process clearly emerges has strong implications regarding the importance of both early identification and subsequent remedial interventions of reading dysfluency and related developmental cognitive functions.

Implications for Remedial Interventions

The critical and interactive roles of specific cognitive and memory functions that facilitate automaticity and early reading skills underscore the importance of a comprehensive investigation of many reading-related cognitive functions, with prereaders and early readers (kindergarten to grade 1), when a diagnosis of potential developmental dyslexia is suspected. There are a number of established and standardized tests that a diagnostician can utilize when investigating prereading capabilities and early reading problems. A thorough assessment for reading deficiencies in prereaders and beginning readers suspected of potential reading problems should include the investigation of developmentally appropriate rapid naming capacities and specific related memory functions, in addition to the assessment of developing phonological awareness capabilities.

A good understanding of the various components of reading fluency skills, and the interactive cognitive processes involved, may provide parents and educators with a broader understanding of the reading process and related reading problems. A solid understanding of those processes can also provide a solid foundation for a better understanding of often used terminologies, enable the most effective assessment techniques, and provide a framework for the most appropriate remedial interventions for each individual.

Once an accurate assessment of early prereading cognitive deficits is obtained, a specific educational diagnostic profile can be established that can then be utilized as a guide for the most appropriate remedial intervention programs for each delayed reader.

Numerous established remedial reading programs focus on the development of automaticity and related reading fluency skills. Special education departments in most school systems will use such standard structured reading programs when a student is determined to need help in reading fluency or is exhibiting early signs of automaticity delays.

CASE STUDY 9.2: LUIS

Luis is a 10-year-old student in the fifth grade with a history of reading difficulties and related academic delays. Despite his recognized academic struggles, first observed in grade 1, Luis has always worked hard in school and wanted to do well academically. Nevertheless, Luis's oral reading has always been notably slow and laborious for his age, and all reading tasks even at his current grade level require additional time allowances. Luis also often has difficulties comprehending what he reads and absorbing information from written text. His teachers over the past several years have observed, however, that if Luis has additional time on reading tasks that allows him to carefully reread information multiple times, his reading comprehension abilities notably increase.

To investigate the underlying causes of his reading concerns, Luis was referred in grade 3 for educational testing by his teacher and his parents. Luis's evaluation process included a comprehensive battery of assessment procedures that included intellectual and cognitive, language, occupational therapy, and academic achievement testing. The cognitive testing indicated that Luis's overall intellectual abilities were within an average range for his age, with strong overall general language reasoning, understanding, and processing, as well as receptive and expressive capabilities. Cognitive strengths were also noted involving learning capacities related to short-term memory and working memory processes.

Cognitive and occupational therapy testing indicated that Luis has neurodevelopmental strengths involving nonverbal and perceptually based reasoning and processing abilities, including overall visual-spatial and visual-perceptual processing capacities. However, this testing also indicated that Luis has significant delays involving speed and efficiency of visual scanning and integrated perceptual and visual-motor functions. Significant delays were also noted involving Luis's ability to automatically and fluently retrieve visual information, a cognitive skill set related to word automaticity capabilities and reading fluency skills.

Academic achievement testing indicated that Luis has a strong foundation of overall phonological processing and memory capabilities. Luis has strong decoding skills and very good applied phonics abilities. Luis's spelling abilities were inconsistent. Significant delays were evident, however, in regard to his reading fluency skills and ability to automatically retrieve the visual codes of words and visual information in general. Luis's reading comprehension abilities were assessed as inconsistent. When he was allowed to read passages repeatedly with no time limits, Luis's comprehension of those materials was good. On timed reading tasks with no opportunities to reread the information, Luis's comprehension was generally quite poor.

Academic testing also provided evidence that Luis has developmentally adequate overall written language abilities, including syntax and grammar structures and general organizational writing skills. He presented specific delays in usage of punctuation. Luis also presented good abilities in math calculation skills and overall applied math knowledge and understanding of concepts and related reasoning principles. He exhibited notable delays, however, involving fluency and the automatic retrieval of mathematical information, such as automatic knowledge of multiplication tables and other math facts.

The assessment data showed that Luis has a reading disability specifically related to automaticity and related word identification skills. Based on assessment and classroom observations, it was understood that even though Luis had good word decoding skills and phonics, he still needed to make the leap from sounding out words when reading to rapidly and automatically retrieving words on sight. Those difficulties affect his ability to read for comprehension and knowledge acquisition, especially when he is required to read quickly and without opportunity to reread.

Based on the assessment process, an IEP was developed for Luis, and implemented throughout all aspects of his educational programming. Luis's IEP provided daily individual and small-group reading instruction. The focus of his remedial reading program was to help him to develop reading fluency and reading comprehension abilities.

Luis's remedial reading program included consistent opportunities and practice utilizing various methods of repeated reading, which facilitates stronger levels of automaticity or fluency. For example, Luis practiced reading passages the first time through for accuracy, with a teacher correcting any errors. He then practiced rereading the same passages to build automaticity and fluency. Related activities involved documenting the time it took Luis to read passages and charting the number of errors to track improvement in reading speed, accuracy, and comprehension. Luis's sight word vocabulary was also increased to improve reading fluency through daily vocabulary practice with flash cards, and frequently reviewing new words. Words that Luis struggled with were documented and reviewed at the beginning and end of each session.

Other remedial strategies included (1) having Luis listen to a teacher read orally or listen to books on tape while he read along, (2) having Luis read new information aloud with his teacher, and (3) encouraging Luis to frequently reread favorite books already familiar to him.

Luis also was provided with weekly individual or small-group remedial instruction to enhance his math fluency skills and his applied knowledge of punctuation rules.

The remedial interventions, instructions, and accommodations that were included in his IEP and the subsequent training and support resulted in Luis making significant and notable gains in math fluency and reading comprehension and written language skills.

READING DISORDERS AND COMPREHENSION DEFICITS

Disorders in reading involve significant impairment in the reading process at many different levels, which typically can involve a range of developmental language processes and functions (Keenan, 2014; Klingner, Vaughn, & Boardman, 2007; Lyons, 2003; Mody & Silliman, 2008a; Vargo et al., 2004). Commonly recognized profiles of reading disabilities may involve deficiencies in applied phonological processes and/or the automatic retrieval of visual information that may subsequently compromise reading at the word level (Peterson & Pennington, 2010; Vargo et al., 2004, 2008; Wolf, 2001). For reading comprehension to expand beyond the word level, however, a complex interaction of language processes and other cognitive functions must occur (Catts & Kamhi, 1999; Jitendra & Gajria, 2011; Klingner, Morrison, & Eppolito, 2011; O'Connor & Vadasy, 2011; Mody & Silliman, 2008b; Vaughn, Swanson, & Solis, 2013; Wallach, Charlton, & Bartholomew, 2014; Windsor & Kohnert, 2008). Within the continuum of reading disabilities is a range of reading problems primarily related to various language-processing deficiencies. Such language-related reading delays span a range of cognitive deficiencies that include various areas and degrees of higher-order language functions and understanding (Catts & Kamhi, 1999; Duke, Cartwright, & Hilden, 2014; Feifer, 2010; Feifer & DeFina, 2000; Lyons, 2003; Mody & Silliman, 2008b; Vaughn et al., 2013; Wallach et al., 2014; Windsor & Kohnert, 2008).

A broad understanding of language functions and disorders, and the relation of such disabilities to certain disorders of reading, is subsequently a critical component of the diagnosis and understanding of the specific nature of an individual's reading deficit.

UNDERSTANDING AND IDENTIFYING LANGUAGE PROCESSING DISABILITIES

Research indicates that reading disabilities involve disorders in areas of the brain that mediate various functions of language and language processing (Shaywitz, 2003). That is why dyslexic individuals, in addition to their reading difficulties, typically also have problems with spelling, expressive writing, word retrieval, and other facets of memory and learning (Feifer & DeFina, 2000, 2002; Spafford & Grosser, 1996).

Throughout the course of the school day, students are immersed in language processes and functions that serve to facilitate all aspects of the educational process. Teachers and students, within the context of interactive teaching and learning, are always and necessarily engaged in communicative interactions. Critical language functions in the classroom that teachers typically utilize can include asking questions pertinent to specific academic content, providing verbal feedback, and even giving specific directions in class or for academic projects. Students are required to utilize integrated higher-order language skills (at appropriate developmental levels) when they perform educational tasks such as giving reports (verbal and/or written), working in student groups, and responding to specific academic content questions. Some academic tasks are of course highly dependent on integrated language skills, such as reading comprehension and writing (Catts & Kamhi, 1999; Fletcher et al., 2007; Spafford & Grosser, 1996). Other academic content areas, such as mathematics, may involve less direct linguistic components, but nevertheless still require good interactive language capabilities and understanding.

The importance of increased language instruction for students with related specific or general deficiencies is evident when considering the amount of research indicating that children with language disorders are much more likely to have delays in academic and social functioning, when compared to non-language-delayed peers (Aram & Nation, 1980; King, Jones, & Laskey, 1982; Kuder, 2003). Concurrently, research clearly indicates that early instruction focused on improving language and communication skills in children relates significantly to increased academic success, especially in the areas of reading (Kuder, 2003; Moats, 2001).

Since a number of reading disability subtypes involve deficiencies in fundamental and higher-order language functions, a comprehensive understanding of language processes is necessary, so that language variables may be considered and effectively investigated in the determination of a possible reading disability profile. The following is a synopsis of information on language functions presented in Chapter 4, that can now be considered in the context of reading comprehension.

THE DEFINITION OF LANGUAGE AND THE FIVE MAJOR LANGUAGE COMPONENTS

Language can be understood as a complex and dynamic system of symbols used for various processes of thinking, reasoning, and communication (Catts & Kamhi, 1999; Kuder, 2003; Stacey, 2003; Singer, 1990; Vargo, 2007). Current understandings of language, based on contemporary societal rules and constructs, posit the following views and positions.

Morphology

While phonology involves the understanding and application of the virtually infinite sound components in language (e.g., such as in the use of phonics skills), what is also necessary for letter-sound combinations to make sense in a language is a set of rules that govern how words are made. Those rules are called morphological rules, and the related language component that governs those rules is known as morphology (Kuder, 2003; Stacey, 2003). Morphology, then, can be thought of as the study of words and how they are formed.

Morphological structures also include prefixes and suffixes used at the beginning and end of words to denote meaning. These elements, known as bound morphemes, have no meaning when used independently. When used in conjunction with various established morphological structures (words), bound morphemes can also be understood as grammatical morphemes that serve specific grammatical and pragmatic functions, and modulate meaning. The components of language that involve aspects of morphology can be complex and extremely important in the understanding of words and written language. The reading process at the understanding and comprehension level can be significantly compromised by deficiencies in the understanding and application of morphologically involved language processing (Rayner & Pollatsek, 1989; Levine, 2002). Difficulties in understanding the meanings of individual words when one is reading, even if those words are accurately decoded, can significantly compromise the process of comprehension (Rayner & Pollatsek, 1989).

Students with a delayed understanding of morphological concepts and constructs are at a disadvantage for developing a strong fund of vocabulary knowledge (Snowling, 2001; Levine, 2002). A good understanding of the various components of morphological processing and awareness, and the linguistic processes involved, may provide parents and educators with a broader understanding of the reading process and reading comprehension problems.

Syntax

Syntax can be understood as language at the sentence level. The established rules of syntax govern sentence organization, word order, and the relationship between words. Syntax regulates how words are combined into larger meaningful units of phrases and sentences. Grammatical structures such as noun and verb phrases are also included in syntactic processes (Akmajian et al., 1988).

Syntax plays a critical role in the understanding and interpretation of grammar and subsequent language meaning (Singer, 1990). Given the depth and complexity of the role of syntax in language processing, neurodevelopmental deficiencies that impact syntactic processing and understanding can compromise the reading comprehension process (Catts & Kamhi, 1999; Rayner & Pollatsek, 1989).

The processing of syntactic information while reading is, at the cognitive level, an automatic process (Rayner & Pollatsek, 1989). That is, a reader will automatically decipher syntax based on an already established and internalized understanding of syntax rules. If a sentence has complex or ambiguous syntax, comprehension can be confused and inaccurate. Due to the automaticity of the processing of syntactic information, readers may often immediately understand sentences inaccurately, and subsequently misread paragraphs and the general meaning of a passage.

Semantics

Semantics is the aspect of language that governs the meanings of words and word combinations (Kuder, 2003; Rayner & Pollatsek, 1989; Singer, 1990). Virtually all languages are rich with words that have multiple meanings, shades of meaning, and contextually driven meanings. The ability to understanding the rich and diverse meanings of a continually expanding vocabulary base is essential to academic success as a student progresses through educational grade levels. Exposure to high numbers of vocabulary words and concepts begins in the early grade school years, peaks again during the high school years, and continues at the college level (Levine, 2002; Singer, 1990).

Students who are neurodevelopmentally delayed in aspects

of semantic processing and understanding are at a disadvantage for acquiring a strong fund of vocabulary knowledge, which in turn facilitates understanding and the acquisition of new knowledge through the reading process and other media (Spafford & Grosser, 1996). A semantically challenged individual in high school typically may have difficulty understanding new words that are being read and subsequently will not effectively learn and incorporate the new knowledge. Knowledge in subject areas such as math and science is often sequential and dependent on the learning and understanding of prior knowledge. Consequently, the student who has not grasped previous knowledge cannot learn additional concepts (Ashcraft, 1989; Matlin, 1989).

Levine (2002) posits that more academically successful students do not necessarily have larger vocabularies than less adept classmates. Rather, students who are more successful in language-related realms tend to have a stronger and more comprehensive understanding of the vocabulary base and word concepts they do possess. Those semantic strengths become even more important as older students encounter words and terms that are conceptually abstract and complex, and the interplay of words and meanings becomes more complicated (e.g., understanding antonyms, synonyms, semantic categories, and similar or ambiguous words and concepts). When considering the importance of semantic variables in the reading and subsequent learning process, it is quite understandable how individuals with neurodevelopmental semantic processing deficiencies are at a significant disadvantage in the classroom and when involved in other learning-related activities. A good understanding of the various components of semantic processing and awareness, and the linguistic processes involved, may provide parents and educators with a broader understanding of the reading process and reading comprehension problems.

Pragmatics

Pragmatics involves the use of language in social and environmental contexts. Listeners (and readers) who are not readily familiar with sociocultural references will simply not have an effective reference point to fill in the meanings that are not literally stated. The ability to effectively apply inference processes while reading narratives is a crucial component for accurate and effective comprehension of written text (Kuder, 2003; Rayner & Pollatsek, 1989; Singer, 1990).

CASE STUDY 9.3: BRAD

Brad is a 15-year-old ninth grader who received special education remedial reading interventions in his elementary grades that focused on improving his reading decoding and fluency skill and his overall writing abilities. Initial cognitive testing at age 10 indicated that Brad's overall intellectual abilities fell within an average range, with inconsistencies noted in areas of language processing involving language reasoning and vocabulary knowledge. Brad's reading abilities at the word level progressively improved throughout his middle school years, and his educational progress and performance were within grade level expectations. As a result, his special education services were discontinued.

In grade 9, due to the increased academic and organizational demands of high school, Brad struggled with most of his classes. He reported and was noted by his teachers as having difficulties with reading comprehension and with lengthy writing tasks and assignments. While Brad always had strong overall math skills and abilities, he began to have difficulties involving multistep word problems. Brad became overwhelmed by the demands of his schoolwork, and by the middle of the academic year he was falling behind in many areas and his overall grades were quite poor.

Brad's evaluation process included a comprehensive battery of assessment procedures that included intellectual and cognitive, language, and academic achievement testing. The cognitive testing showed overall intellectual abilities within an average range for his age, with strengths in nonverbal and perceptually based reasoning and processing abilities, including overall visual-spatial and visual-perceptual processing capacities, and visual scanning and integrated visual-perceptual and visual-motor functions. Brad also had strengths in automatically and fluently retrieving visual information, a cognitive skill set related to word automaticity and reading fluency skills. Cognitive strengths were also noted in short-term memory and working memory processes.

Cognitive and extended language testing revealed developmental delays and deficits in many aspects of language processing and understanding, including language reasoning, vocabulary, semantic and pragmatic language, and contextual language.

Academic achievement testing indicated that Brad has a strong foundation of fundamental reading skills involving word decoding, word identification, and reading fluency. He also demonstrated good math calculation and fluency skills. Delays were noted, however, in his reading comprehension abilities and reasoning capabilities in the context of mathematical word problems. Brad did demonstrate adequate writing skills and knowledge when he was required to write brief sentences or paragraphs, such as understanding and usage of basic grammar structures and punctuation rules. When required to generate lengthier and more conceptually complex examples of written text, Brad's writing abilities were notably delayed.

The assessment data provided strong and consistent evidence that Brad has a language-based learning disability that is also resulting in a reading disability. Based on the assessment processes, an IEP was developed for Brad and implemented throughout all aspects of his educational programming. He was provided with intensive remedial language instruction twice a week in school, with a focus on improving his applied understanding of language reasoning concepts, vocabulary and word knowledge and usage, and semantic, pragmatic, and contextual language. That instruction emphasized the use and understanding of those higher-order language areas in the context of many academic content areas and tasks, such as reading comprehension and written language.

Brad's IEP provided daily individual and small-group reading instruction. The focus of his remedial reading program was to help him develop and acquire appropriate reading comprehension strategies and abilities. The remedial reading program included various reading comprehension strategies, including asking what the goal of reading is, how to read for different purposes and with different materials, and how to monitor one's reading processes to facilitate comprehension and acquisition of information. Brad was also taught how to develop and use reading comprehension tools such as outlines and summaries of readings, and various graphic organizers.

It was determined by his educational team that Brad's reading disability would likely impede his access to grade-level texts and readings. Thus, whenever possible and appropriate Brad was provided with modified texts and class handouts to bypass his reading difficulties and to help him more efficiently access the information being taught across academic content areas.

To address his writing difficulties, Brad's educational plan included the following interventions and accommodations. He received weekly individual or small-group instruction in using a systematic process approach to writing, which included a series of steps such as brainstorming, organizing ideas into an outline or graphic representation, writing a first draft based on an outline, and generating multiple edits in the process of finalizing a written narrative.

Brad's course grades across all academic areas were based on his knowledge and understanding of course materials, and not on the writing assignments for those courses. He received weekly training in the use of word processing programs, with a focus on tools such as grammar, spell check, and cut-and-paste" functions in organizational writing contexts.

To address his math difficulties related to his language disability, Brad was taught alternate and multiple ways to analyze and solve math problems, especially word problems. For instance, Brad was taught extended math vocabularies to help him understand what a word problem is asking for and to more effectively identify common types of math questions by analyzing the language or form of the problem. Brad was also taught various math problem-solving templates with step-by-step guidelines he could follow once he identified what a particular math problem required.

ENHANCING READING COMPREHENSION ABILITIES IN CLASSROOMS

It has been shown that student communications can be improved in the classroom with the use of various teaching formats that strongly involve interactive language processes, which subsequently facilitates improved language knowledge and functioning (Berninger & Wolf, 2009; Daly, Chafouleas, & Skinner, 2005;

Klingner et al., 2007; Kuder, 2003). One general model proposed by Dudley-Marling and Searle (1988) includes the following three teaching suggestions to enhance classroom communication:

1. The physical setting (the classroom) should by design help to promote and encourage talking and interactive communication, including reading-related activities. For instance, small work centers, circular tables, and so on, can be used when appropriate and possible.
2. When possible, a teacher should provide ample opportunities for students to use language and communicate during reading and learning processes. For example, verbal communication on an academic topic can actually be considered a goal of a given lesson.
3. A teacher should provide opportunities for students to use language for a variety of purposes and audiences in reading activities; for example, sharing personal examples related to academic topics with peers and adults (parents).

Klingner and colleagues (2007) presented a range of language-involved teaching and learning strategies for students that enable stronger reading comprehension abilities and related general conceptual understanding of information from written language:

1. Techniques for formulating main ideas and summarizing written information
2. Techniques for understanding and formulating main ideas from sections of written texts and narratives
3. Story retelling techniques in verbal dialogue contexts to help formulate summarization of written materials and stories

4. Reciprocal teaching techniques to help facilitate comprehension that include various components of classroom dialogue and cognitive scaffolding teaching techniques

Daly and colleagues (2005) outlined other proven valuable teaching and studying strategies especially helpful to older students with reading comprehension and related language processing difficulties to help facilitate good understanding of written text:

1. Prereading a story for grammar understanding and clarification
2. Providing students with outlines and study guides on written materials, both before and after actual reading activities
3. Teaching reading- and language-challenged students effective and alternative note-taking strategies to help clarify understanding and comprehension of written information

Swanson (2009) posited a common conceptual core of instructions to provide a combination of learning and studying tools and strategies to learners with comprehension difficulties, including the following:

1. Initially stating learning objectives and orienting students to what they will be learning and what will be expected of them.
2. Initially repeating techniques and skills to help students understand information being obtained through reading and all information processing modalities.
3. As information is being presented or read, teachers can repeatedly give examples to provide enhanced understanding of concepts and information.

4. While information is being presented or read, teachers can pose related questions (cognitive probes) to assess both levels of understanding and possible misunderstanding of topic information.

5. Using frequent assessment procedures with immediate feedback to assess student understanding and facilitate comprehension and conceptual learning.

Chapter 10

SPECIFIC LEARNING DISORDERS IN WRITTEN LANGUAGE

The invention and development of written language in its earliest form of cuneiform symbols dates back approximately 5,000 years, with more structured writing systems evolving over the past few thousand years (Berninger & Wolf, 2009; Wolf, 2007). In the modern world, the acquisition and use of writing skills and functional written language is a core component of educational processes and requirements, across all grade levels (elementary through postsecondary) and academic areas (Berninger & Richards, 2002; Stone et al., 2014; Zemelman et al., 2005).

From a neurodevelopmental perspective, written language involves an acquired set of academic skills, which include a complex combination of cognitive functions and neurodevelopmental constructs (Berninger & Richards, 2002; Chittooran & Tait, 2005;Feifer & DeFina, 2002; Hale & Fiorello, 2004). Since writing at all levels involves a range of neurodevelopmental functions and related cognitive processes, the various subtypes of disorders of written language likely have multiple etiologies that involve biological, genetic, environmental, and psychosocial factors (Fletcher et al., 2007). Consider that writing at all grade levels requires motor functions (handwriting and computer keyboard) and the utilization of integrated applied understandings of multiple language functions. Indeed, applied knowledge of syntax, semantics, spelling, vocabulary and word understanding, and virtually all language-related functions come into play in writing processes and contexts (American Psychiatric Association, 2013; Berninger & Richards, 2002; Berninger et al., 2009; Feifer & DeFina, 2002). Developmentally adequate cognitive functions involving spatial processing and awareness and sequential processing abilities are necessary in writing contexts, as well as organizational abilities, aspects of attention regulation, and various executive functions (Feifer & DeFina, 2002; Levine, 2002b). Components of memory functions, such as working memory abilities and automatic memory capacities, also are utilized in writing (Berninger, 2008; Berninger & Richards, 2002; Feifer & DeFina, 2002). Processes of written language, in addition to integrated language functions, also are closely related to various areas of reading and oral language (Berninger, 2010; Wallach et al., 2014). It has also been shown that individuals with written language disorders may also have difficulties with math processes that involve written output, such as in mathematical word problems (Berninger, 2010).

A disorder in an area of written language is also known as dysgraphia, a word with Greek roots that means "impaired" (the prefix *dys*) and the base word *graph*, which translates to "letter-form produced by hand" (Berninger, 2010). Disorders of written language, which can also then be diagnostically described as dysgraphia, can therefore be understood as developmentally delayed writing abilities and skills (American Psychiatric Association, 2013; Feifer & DeFina, 2002). It is important to note that there are various subtypes of writing disability, based on the areas of cognitive and neurodevelopmental deficits that underlie the writing delays (Berninger, 2010; Berninger & Wolf, 2009; Berninger et al., 2009; Chittooran & Tait, 2005; Feifer & DeFina, 2002).

CASE STUDY 10.1 JASMINE

Jasmine is a 10 year old fourth grader who has been receiving special education services in occupational therapy since grade two to address developmental delays in fine-motor functions. She also was recognized as having developmental reading delays in grade two, for which she received additional weekly reading instructions in a small group setting within the context of her school system's Response to Intervention (RTI) remedial model for addressing students with recognized academic delays. Jasmine's abilities in her fine-motor functions and related tasks involving integrated finger and hand coordination did show improvement in grades two and three, but were still an area of concern for her by the beginning of grade four. In grade two, Jasmine was observed to have notable problems forming letter shapes, her spacing between letters and words was developmentally poor, she evidenced limited understandings and usage of uppercase and lower case letters and related grammatical rules, and she typically had difficulties writing and drawing in lines and margins at a grade appropriate level. Jasmine's handwriting delays were also evident in her performances on various math related tasks. For instance, Jasmine appeared to have a strong developing sense of applied conceptual mathematical knowledge and understanding of sequential processes involved in math calculation solving. She had consistent problems, however, accurately aligning columns and rows of number such as in addition and division problems, and those difficulties over time appeared to compromise the development and progress of Jasmine's overall mathematical skills and knowledge.

Jasmine's pencil grip when writing and drawing was noticed by her second grade teacher and occupational therapist to be awkward and quite ineffective, and those developmental concerns were addressed in her ongoing occupational therapy programming.

By the end of grade three and the beginning of grade four, Jasmine's handwriting and related skills such as drawing and coloring were still developmentally delayed. When she engaged in lengthier writing related tasks in her various class subjects and activities, Jasmine's handwriting at times was virtually illegible. It was noted by her teacher early in grade four that Jasmine's handwriting reflected developmentally delayed combinations and usage of combined print and cursive words, and she frequently omitted words in sentences that she likely did initially mentally formulate and intended to write but then did not actually write down. By the beginning of grade four, Jasmine's writing reflected delayed understandings and usages of developing syntax, grammar structure, and punctuation rules. Her expressive written language skills overall were observably much poorer than Jasmine's expressive *oral* language abilities.

Her third and fourth grade teachers believed that Jasmine's overall reading skills were at least developmentally adequate, and in fact her reading support services were discontinued for her at the end of grade three. Her oral reading fluency with grade level texts was never noted by those teachers as problematic, and throughout the third grade Jasmine presented no concerns involving her sight word acquisition and vocabulary. In the earlier months of grade four, however, Jasmine's teacher observed and documented that Jasmine was presenting increasing difficulties in her reading comprehension abilities, especially when she was required in class and with homework to read lengthier amounts of texts and narratives to access and obtain academic content information.

Given her continuing academic difficulties and delays,

Jasmine was referred for a comprehensive psycho-educational evaluation by her fourth grade teacher and her parents. That evaluation included intellectual and cognitive testing, a comprehensive speech and language evaluation, updated occupational therapy, and academic achievement testing. The information obtained from her cognitive testing provided consistent indications that Jasmine's overall intellectual abilities were within an average range, and that she also had above average range learning strengths in cognitive areas involving non-verbal reasoning abilities and visual-spatial and visual-perceptual processing. Significant developmental delays were noted, however, in regard to Jasmine's speed and efficiency of integrated visual-motor processing and functions.

Based on the information obtained from her cognitive testing and her comprehensive speech and language evaluation, it was recognized that Jasmine was also a student with significant language processing developmental delays. Her assessed areas of language deficits involved general language reasoning capacities and understanding of higher-language concepts such as semantic language, contextual language, inferential language, social-pragmatic language, and applied understandings of vocabulary and language ambiguities. In other words, Jasmine was a student with average range overall intellectual abilities with a specific language based learning disability and a concurrent learning disability in written language.

The occupational therapy component of her evaluation indicated that Jasmine also still had neurodevelopmental delays involving her integrated fine-motor functions. Even with the remedial interventions that she received in her earlier elementary grades, Jasmine still had neurologically based delays that interfered with physical skill areas such as handwriting and other tasks involving integrated fine-motor skills.

Jasmine's academic achievement testing showed that she was academically strong in her word identification and reading fluency skills. She presented, however, moderate delays in her word decoding skills when reading unfamiliar words, and significant academic deficits involving her reading comprehension capacities. Jasmine's assessed achievement levels in written language were quite delayed. More specifically, she exhibited deficits in all assessed areas of writing, including her applied knowledge of syntax and grammar rules and structures, her knowledge and application of punctuation rules, her spelling, vocabulary knowledge and usage in writing contexts, and her developing general organizational writing capabilities. Academic achievement testing further indicated that Jasmine had developmentally strong applied conceptual math knowledge and understanding, but she presented inconsistencies in her math calculations skills and knowledge.

As a result of the findings of her psycho-educational assessment and her observed ongoing academic difficulties, an Individualized Educational Plan (IEP) was developed and implemented for Jasmine, which included a very comprehensive program of special education services for her. Her Individualized Educational Plan included multiple remedial interventions and supports and accommodations in areas involving language and language arts, and specific instructions and supports for reading comprehension and all aspects of written language. Some specifics of the special education services that Jasmine received are as follows:

Jasmine received extensive remedial speech and language services in a small group language LD program that met several times a week and progressively covered all aspects of language in the primary contexts of educational applications across all academic disciplines. For instance, Jasmine's instructions in language areas involving her understanding of syntax and vocabulary were consistently practiced and reinforced in her remedial writing instructions and school-based writing activities. Her instructions involving more abstract and higher-order language concepts such as the understanding of semantic and pragmatic language, contextual language, metaphorical language, and inferential language were taught and practiced in the contexts of reading for comprehension, understanding, and meaning.

Jasmine received weekly remedial instructions in written language in a small group writing class with a special education teacher. Her remedial writing instructions were systematically integrated with Jasmine's ongoing special education language classes, to better ensure and reinforce language concepts and knowledge in the context of written language and general language arts.

To address complexity of writing involving all aspects of organization and implementation of written text and narrative, Jasmine's remedial writing training also focused on her developing a systematic "process" approach to writing. To that end, Jasmine was taught and allowed ample opportunities to practice how to develop and generate initial drafts of writing based on a primary general outline, and she was taught and encouraged to practice and use various techniques to allow her to "brainstorm" ideas and then systematically organize written information into outlines and various forms of graphic representations. Jasmine was also progressively taught and allowed to practice a range of sequential and organizational writing strategies that helped her to more effectively break down writing tasks and assignments into organized and manageable steps, and allowed for more systematic ways of developing and utilizing multiple and sequential edits when writing for organization of ideas, content, grammar, syntax, punctuation, and spelling. Consistent feedback was provided to Jasmine by her teachers in all of those learned areas, and consistently reinforced in the contexts of her daily classroom work and her homework.

To address the volume of writing required of Jasmine on a daily basis in school and the difficulties she encountered when writing, all measures of academic content knowledge for Jasmine that utilized any writing tasks (such as tests and classroom learning activities) excluded various grading criteria such as spelling and good letter formation, and generally allowed for a primary focus on most of Jasmine's acquisition of academic content information and knowledge.

To address rate of writing involving her speed and efficiency on writing tasks, Jasmine's teachers allowed her extended time allowances whenever possible on all academic tasks involving any aspect of written language, including all classwork homework, and longer-term and extended projects that included any writing.

Given her fine-motor and visual-motor deficits that compromise her physical writing capabilities, Jasmine was provided with individualized computer keyboarding skill training and allowed to use computer keyboard/typing formats whenever possible for academic tasks involving writing.

Jasmine was also provided with instructions and training in the applied knowledge and use of word processing programs, with a specific focus on learning and utilizing various writing tools common in word processing such as "cut and paste" and "spell check" functions. When it was not possible or appropriate for Jasmine to use a computer when writing and she needed to write by hand, Jasmine was allowed to use writing tools that she was most comfortable with and that best allowed her to write efficiently and effectively, such as erasable pens and pens with large grips.

Whenever possible and appropriate, Jasmine was offered

alternative methods for preventing her classwork and homework and to demonstrate mastery of knowledge and concepts across various academic disciplines. For instance, Jasmine often offered the option of utilizing oral tests instead of written tests, and she was encouraged when appropriate to present oral presentations in class.

PROCESSES THAT CAN INHIBIT WRITING DEVELOPMENT

As students progress through school, they are increasingly expected to express what they know about many different subjects through writing. If a child fails to develop foundational writing skills in earlier grades, he or she may consequently lack writing speed, fluency, and applied higher-order language skill sets required in developing writing processes as learning demands increase over time. For a student who experienced poor early writing development and continues to struggle with writing problems and delays, the writing process itself can interfere with educational functioning and progress across many academic areas (Berninger et al., 2009; Levine, 1995, 1998, 2002b).

CASE STUDY 10.2 EVAN

Evan is a 16 year old student in the 11th grade, with a previous diagnosis of Attention Deficit Hyperactivity Disorder and related learning difficulties involving organizational and executive functions including some aspects of memory and information processing. Evan was diagnosed with his attention disorder at age twelve, and he has been prescribed medication interventions for that diagnosis since that time to the present, with reported generally positive results.

When Evan was suspected of having an attentional disorder by his school system and his parents, he underwent a comprehensive neuropsychological and educational evaluation as part of the diagnostic process. That evaluation documented that Evan was a student with above average range overall intellectual abilities and excellent learning capacities involving overall language and non-language based reasoning and processing. The evaluation also documented, however, that Evan was a student with neurodevelopmental deficits in many facets of learning and memory as well as in related areas of abilities described and understood as executive functions. The academic achievement component of his neurodevelopmental evaluation documented that Evan had very strong academic skills involving all aspects of reading and math. His overall assessed writing skills were within an average range, with some inconsistencies not in regard to organizational writing skills.

Based on his diagnosis of Attention Deficit Hyperactivity Disorder and his recognition of having related processing and executive function deficits, Evan's school system developed an educational accommodation plan that was implemented and followed throughout all of his school day and across all educational activities. Evan's educational accommodations, which continued into his high school grades, were instrumental in his overall academic success through his middle school grades and early high school years.

As Evan progressed into grade eleven, the increased organizational and academic demands resulted in his falling behind in his studies and his course work. Evan's performance across academic areas started to become notably inconsistent, and his grades began to fall. Of most concern by his teachers was Evan's progressive difficulties with academic tasks involving written language and writing in general. Evan did seek out after school help from several language arts teachers, and those educators noted that Evan had a number of difficulties that were obvious when he was endeavoring to express himself through writing.

Some of his most salient writing problems involved inconsistent use of correct grammar and syntax structures most noted on longer narratives and writing assignments, inconsistent use of punctuation rules, difficulties organizing and monitoring his thoughts in the writing process. All of his teachers that included writing activities and assignments in their classes described Evan as an intelligent and hardworking student with insufficient writing skills for his grade level and poor overall organizational abilities

As a result of his decreasing academic performances and subsequent concerns of his teachers and parents, Evan underwent an updated educational evaluation, which included cognitive and academic achievement testing. The cognitive component of that assessment documented that Evan's general intellectual and learning profile was consistent with his previous neuropsychological evaluation at age twelve. That is, he was again found to be a student with overall intellectual abilities within an above average range who also had learning difficulties involving memory and executive functions. The updated evaluation also documented that Evan's overall reading and math skills and knowledge remained strong. His overall written language abilities, primarily in areas related to aspects of organizational writing, were considerably below grade level.

Based on the findings of the updated educational evaluation, Evan's school system developed and implemented a program of special education services for him. Within the context of an Individualized Educational Plan, Evan began to receive ongoing remedial instructions in all areas of organizational writing and planning. In addition, Evan also received ongoing instructions that progressively taught him a range of organizational and studying strategies, and he was assisted by his special education teachers in consistently using those newly acquired strategies and skills in all of his classes.

In Chapter 2, various neurodevelopmental constructs were outlined, with examples of the impact those neurocognitive functions can have on learning and learning performance. There is ample evidence of how writing functions and written language abilities can be compromised in many ways by deficits in neurodevelopmental constructs (Berninger, 2010; Berninger & Wolf, 2009; Berninger et al., 2009; Chittooran & Tait, 2005; Englert et al., 2009; Glatthorn et al., 2009).

Levine (1998, 2002b) has documented how multiple neurodevelopmental constructs support virtually all levels of writing, and how deficits in various neurodevelopmental processes can negatively impact writing abilities and writing development. Feifer and DeFina (2002) provide extensive outlines and explanations of the impact of neurocognitive deficits on various aspects of writing processes. The following related overviews draw on information provided primarily by Levine (1998) in his book *Developmental Variation and Learning Disorders*, and Feifer and DeFina (2002) in their book *The Neuropsychology of Written Language Disorders*.

Attention Deficits and Disorders

In written language, students with attentional regulation difficulties may:

- Have difficulties initiating and continuing writing assignments
- Have inconsistent levels of writing legibility and general output
- Have poorly organized writing due to deficient self-monitoring
- Have many careless writing errors due to deficient self-monitoring
- Have inconsistent spelling, grammar structures, and punctuation

- Have mental fatigue or tiredness while writing and ultimate lack of persistence
- Have inconsistent and uneven memory functions

Language Deficits and Disorders

In written language, students with language disabilities may:

- Have difficulties with sentence structure and word order
- Have delayed vocabulary knowledge and applications
- Use developmentally simplistic sentence structures
- Have difficulty with word sounds, spelling, and meanings
- Have ineffective referencing and narrative cohesion
- Use contextual and colloquial language ineffectively
- Have trouble utilizing reading back written text as an editing strategy

Memory Deficits and Disorders

In written language, students with language disabilities may:

- Have poor recall of applied vocabulary knowledge
- Have poor recall of applied spelling patterns and rules
- Have poor recall of capitalization and punctuation rules
- Have poor recall of grammar rules
- Have weak word retrieval capabilities
- Have an inconsistent flow of thinking

Temporal-Sequential Ordering Deficits and Disorders

In written language, students with temporal-sequential ordering deficits may:

- Have developmentally poor letter formation
- Have transposed letters and spelling omissions
- Have poor narrative sequencing
- Have developmentally poor theme transitions

- Have developmentally poor writing cohesiveness
- Have developmentally poor writing organization and output

Spatial Ordering Deficits and Disorders

In written language, students with spatial ordering deficits may:

- Have uneven spacing between letters and words
- Use lines and margins ineffectively
- Have poor or disorganized spatial page planning
- Have deficient visualization of words and letters
- Have general visual organization difficulties

Neuromotor Deficits and Disorders

In written language, students with neuromotor deficits, especially in the form of graphomotor delays, may:

- Have slow and laborious handwriting
- Produce a developmentally limited amount of writing
- Have poor writing legibility
- Have an awkward or inefficient pencil grasp
- Have a developmentally poor lack of written fluency
- May write developmentally slowly and with great effort
- May have a preference for printing
- May find it hard to form letters
- May typically write only very short passages when required to write by hand

Higher-Order Cognition and Language Deficits and Disorders

In written language, students with higher-order cognition and language deficits may:

- Have difficulty developing, organizing, and expanding ideas

- Have difficulties with the written development of abstract ideas
- Have difficulty with writing tasks that require creativity or critical thinking
- Present developmentally simple and concrete ideas
- Have weak position and opinion development
- Have poor audience awareness
- Typically only generate developmentally limited written output when required

Executive Function Deficits and Disorders

In written language, students with executive function deficits may:

- Have overall poor organizational writing skills
- Have poor idea generation
- Often develop poorly organized sentences and paragraphs
- Often perseverate on a theme and shift ideas poorly
- Have poor planning abilities in writing construction and development
- Have poor self-monitoring and editing abilities
- Adequately initiate a writing activity but have difficulty completing it

Chapter 11

SPECIFIC LEARNING DISORDERS IN MATH

A specific learning disability in mathematics, known as dyscalculia, refers to a wide range of learning disabilities involving various aspects of mathematics. There is no single type of math disability, as specific learning disorders in mathematics can vary in many ways and subsequently affect people differently across grade levels and later across stages of life (Agaliotis, 2009; Barkley, 1997, 1998; Dawson & Guare, 2004; Emerson & Babtie, 2010; Henderson, 2012; Levine, 1998, 2002a, 2002b; Lyon & Krasnegor, 1996; Montague & Jitendra, 2006; Pennington, 2009; Sousa, 2008).

Math disabilities or dyscalculia can be further understood as difficulties and deficits in the ability to process mathematical information involving an applied understanding of number sense, memorization of arithmetic facts, fluent and accurate math calculation processes, and accurate mathematical reasoning (American Psychiatric Association, 2013; Berninger & Richards, 2002; Barnes et al., 2010; Fletcher et al., 2007).

Although definitions of dyscalculia do vary, it is generally agreed that a specific learning disability in mathematics is a neurologically based disorder that originates as a genetic or congenital disorder of the brain and causes a discrepancy between an individual's general cognitive level and mathematical abilities. As such, math disabilities of all variations can be considered neurodevelopmental disorders (Geary, 2000; Rourke & Conway, 1997; Wadlington & Wadlington, 2008).

Disorders of mathematics are also commonly related to and often exist with other learning disabilities and neurodevelopmental disorders, including dyslexia or disorders of reading, dysgraphia or disorders of written language, and language-based learning disabilities, motor disorders, and attention deficit disorders (Miller, 2010a; Miles & Miles, 1992; Spafford & Grosser, 1996; Wadlington & Wadlington, 2008; Yeo, 2005).

While there is a range of neurodevelopmental and related cognitive constructs that can contribute to delays and deficits in mathematics, it has been shown that there are two major areas of cognitive weakness that generally contribute to specific learning disabilities in math: (1) visual-spatial difficulties, which may result in a person having trouble visually processing information; and (2) language processing difficulties on many levels, from phonological processing to higher-order language understanding (Emerson & Babtie, 2010; Henderson, 2012; Levine, 1998, 2002a, 2002b; Miles & Miles, 1992).

CASE STUDY 11.1 HELENA

Helena is a 14 year old eighth grader who was referred for an educational evaluation by her math teacher and her parents because of difficulties over the past academic year involving Helena's performance and progress primarily in her math classes, but also to some degree in other classes that involved extensive written assignments and tests and more long-term writing and research. Helena has had previously noted difficulties in math during her elementary school years, but not in any areas involving language arts. Her past observed math difficulties, beginning in grade four, were noted in areas involving effectively using margins and lines when organizing and solving number problems (such as in addition and subtraction equations), poor and disorganized visual planning of math and number problems, the production of uneven spacing and planning in the processes of writing out math calculations and math word problems, notable difficulties with any math related activities involving the visual awareness and mental manipulation of visual-spatial information such as in fundamental geometric concepts, and in general poor math calculation skills.

To address those academic concerns, Helena underwent a special evaluation assessment process, which included cognitive and academic achievement testing, and an occupational therapy evaluation. The cognitive component from that assessment process indicated that Helena had overall intellectual abilities within an average range of functioning, with *above average* range overall cognitive abilities involving language based areas of learning, reasoning, processing, and understanding. Her fourth grade assessment, however, also indicated that Helena was an individual with a range of cognitive weaknesses that were mostly within low average range functioning for her age. Those weaknesses and developmental delays involved areas such as visual-spatial and visual-perceptual processing and awareness, and speed and efficiency of visual-perceptual processing and integrated visual-motor functions and visual-association capacities.

Her fourth grade academic achievement assessment also indicated that at that time Helena was academically delayed in her general math calculation skills and knowledge and her applied conceptual math abilities especially involving the organization and strategic solving of mathematical word problems. Helena was noted, however, to have developmentally strong math capacities involving her ability to automatically retrieve visual and verbal math facts, such as in efficiently knowing time table facts.

The academic components of the fourth grade testing

also indicated that Helena had strong fundamental reading abilities at the word reading levels, which included good word identification and reading fluency skills, and solid word decoding capabilities when she encountered unfamiliar words. Moderate weaknesses were noted, however, involving Helena's reading comprehension abilities. In regard to further language arts areas of learning, the testing indicated that Helena's overall written language skills and knowledge were developmentally adequate. Her writing strengths were noted in areas such as the applied understanding of language based syntax, grammar structure, and punctuation rules and knowledge in writing contexts. Marginal weaknesses were noted involving Helena's developing organizational writing skills and knowledge.

The occupational therapy evaluation indicated that Helena was not developmentally delayed in any of the assessed areas fine-motor functions. There were moderate delays evident, however, in regard to her general gross-motor functioning, especially involving balance and physical body awareness. The occupational therapy examiner documented that those assessed areas of delay could impact on Helena's ability to successfully participate and master physically related activities such as various sports (especially sports requiring excellent balance and eye-hand coordination) and expressive dancing (which Helena had an interest in pursuing).

Based on the assessment findings from her fourth grade educational evaluation, which included a consideration of her past and recent academic difficulties, Helena was diagnosed as having a specific learning disability in mathematics. The educational team also considered the possibility that Helena was also a student with a nonverbal disability, or at least elements of that cognitive profile. While the information obtained from her intellectual and cognitive assessment (very strong global language based learning abilities in contrast to moderately delayed overall perceptually based cognitive capabilities) did reflect at least possible components of a nonverbal learning disability, that diagnosis was tabled and considered to be specifically assessed at another time. Helena's assessed learning problems in math were addressed with special education interventions involving an Individualized Educational Plan that focused on remedial interventions in all areas of applied mathematical skills and knowledge. Helena's special education interventions in math resulted in her making progressive gains in her general math skills and knowledge in grade four through six, and those services and her IEP were discontinued for her by the end of her sixth grade of studies.

As a result of Helena's recent academic concerns, she underwent updated cognitive and academic achievement testing by her school system to investigate the possible need for re-establishing remedial academic interventions and supports for her at that time. The more recent cognitive assessment reflected a very similar profile as Helena's previous intellectual assessment, with very strong general language based learning capabilities in contrast to moderately delayed areas of visual-spatial and visual-perceptually based processing. Her updated academic achievement testing in grade eight indicated that Helena has developmentally adequate math calculation skills and knowledge, but her ability to solve math word problems was notably delayed. Helena's ability to mathematically understand and problem solve geometric concepts were a particular area of mathematical difficulty for her. Achievement testing in her eighth grade also reflected academic delays in reading comprehension and in organizational writing abilities.

Based on the assessment findings from her eighth grade educational evaluation, which included a consideration of her recent academic difficulties, Helena was again diagnosed as having a specific learning disability in mathematics, along with specific learning disabilities in reading comprehension and organizational writing. Another Individualized Educational Plan was developed and special educational interventions and supports were established for her. Helena's eighth grade Individual Educational Plan involved weekly remedial math and written language instructions in small group formats of two to four students, included the following components:

Helena was provided with specific instructions involving visually organizing more complex math calculation problems typically encountered at the middle school level, such as multiple row long division and multiplication. She received extensive remedial training in regard to understanding math word problems and following templates of sequences of steps to solve all math calculations and problems.

Helena was taught and encouraged to practice alternate and multiple ways to analyze and solve math problems, especially in the context of mathematical word problems. Helena was taught extended math vocabularies to better help her to understand what a word problem is asking for and to more effectively identify common types of math questions by analyzing the language or form of the problem.

Helena was provided with remedial reading instructions in a small group that involved teaching her various reading comprehension strategies, with a specific focus on effectively utilizing those learned strategies in solving math word problems. Some of the educational and learning strategies that Helena was progressively taught, practiced, and reinforced in her math classes included self-monitoring strategies when reading for comprehension, and how to generate and successfully use comprehension tools such as summaries, highlighting, outlines, and graphic representations.

Helena's Individualized Educational Plan also included weekly small group instructions which focused on her developing stronger organizational writing skills, and the application of those abilities for the solving of math word problems as well as in all academic areas that required lengthy and well-organized writing and related planning activities.

Given Helena's assessed perceptually based developmental delays and related cognitive processing deficits, the following recommendations/accommodations were implemented for her across all of her educational environments and experiences, and especially in her math and language arts classes:

All visual material presented to Helena in her math classes were simple in format and uncluttered by excessive visual information.

Whenever possible in her math classes, Helena was assisted in planning and organizing assigned tasks by providing visual cues (e.g., numbering lines; designated "boxes in which to work; etc.).

Dyscalculia has also been divided into subtypes in various ways (Wadlington & Wadlington, 2008). For instance, Geary (2000) developed the following useful categorization involving various neurodevelopmental aspects of memory, which include the following:

- Semantic memory, which could impact math functions such as difficulties retrieving arithmetic facts
- Procedural memory, which could impact math functions such as understanding and applying mathematical procedures
- Visuospatial memory, which could impact math functions such as spatially represented numerical information including columns, place values, or geometry

WARNING SIGNS OF MATH DISABILITIES

Having trouble learning math skills does not necessarily mean a person has a learning disability, as individuals commonly learn math at a different pace. Developmental variations and functioning should always be considered in all learning processes, including the teaching and learning of mathematics (Emerson & Babtie, 2010; Henderson, 2012; Levine, 1998, 2002a, 2002b). The U.S. National Center for Learning Disabilities (2014) outlines a range of developmental expectations and related potential indications of a math disability for educators and parents to use as a guide when math-related learning disabilities are suspected, based on general age and developmental standards (Table 11.1).

TABLE 11.1 WARNING SIGNS OF MATH DISABILITIES BY AGE

In Young Children (Preschool to Kindergarten)	In Elementary and Middle School-Aged Children	In Adolescents and Adults
• Difficulty learning to count • Trouble recognizing printed numbers • Difficulty tying together the idea of a number • Poor memory for numbers • Trouble organizing things in a logical way (e.g., putting round objects in one place and square ones in another)	• Trouble learning math facts (addition, subtraction, multiplication, division) • Difficulty developing math problem-solving skills • Poor long-term memory for math functions • Not familiar with math vocabulary • Difficulty measuring things • Avoiding games that require strategy	• Difficulty estimating costs such as grocery bills • Difficulty learning math concepts beyond the basic math facts • Poor ability to budget or balance a checkbook • Trouble with concepts of time, such as sticking to a schedule or approximating time • Trouble with mental math • Difficulty finding different approaches to one problem

CASE STUDY 11.2 JARED

Jared is a 16 year old tenth grade student with a previous diagnosis of Attention Deficit Hyperactivity Disorder. Jared's attentional difficulties have been recognized since his elementary grades, and he has been prescribed medication interventions since for attentional control that have been consistently beneficial to him. In grades three and four, Jared's attentional difficulties were noted by his teachers to interfere with his academic functioning and progress. As a result, his school system conducted an educational evaluation for Jared when he was in grade four, which included cognitive and academic achievement testing, and attention rating scales completed by his classroom teacher. The academic achievement component of his fourth grade educational assessment indicated that at that time Jared was a student with developmentally strong basic reading skills and reading comprehension abilities, grade appropriate developing written language skills and knowledge, and average range applied conceptual math and math calculation capabilities. The cognitive component of the fourth grade assessment indicated that Jared's overall intellectual abilities fell within an above average range, and that he had excellent overall language and non-language based reasoning and processing learning strengths and developmentally strong integrated visual-motor capacities. The information obtained from the teacher attention rating scale supported concerns for Jared regarding significant attentional problems.

Jared's educational assessment was reviewed by his educational team and his pediatrician. While he was not found by his school system to have a specific learning disability, the assessment information was an important consideration for his pediatrician in the determination of a diagnosis for Jared of Attention Deficit Hyperactivity Disorder.

Based on that diagnosis, educational accommodations to address his attentional concerns were established for Jared across all of his academic settings, which continued throughout his elementary and middle school years.

When Jared began high school at grade nine, the increased academic and organizational demands of the higher grade levels resulted in him again having notable academic difficulties. Jared was observed in a number of his classes to have problems involving his planning and organization of homework and long-term assignments, as well as in regard to his organizational writing skills in all of his ninth and tenth grade classes that involved written expression on assignments and tests. Of most concern was Jared's poor academic performance in his past three math classes. While Jared overall did well academically in math during his later elementary and middle school grades, his ninth and tenth grade math classes became increasingly difficult for him.

Given his educational concerns in high school, Jared was referred for another educational assessment which included updated intellectual/cognitive testing and academic achievement testing, as well as a neurodevelopmental assessment component to obtain information regarding more specific aspects of Jared's learning, memory, and executive function capabilities. The cognitive and neurodevelopmental aspects of his tenth grade testing indicated, consistent with previous educational testing, that Jared was a student with above average range overall intellectual and general language based learning capabilities. That updated testing also documented that Jared was a student with neurodevelopmental delays in a number of cognitive areas involving learning and memory functions and related cognitive/information processing abilities, as well as in areas of learning involving applied organizational capabilities and multiple executive functions. It was noted by Jared's educational team that difficulties and developmental delays in areas of memory and executive functions are very typical in individuals with Attention Deficit Hyperactivity Disorder, which Jared had previously been diagnosed with and medically treated for.

The updated academic achievement testing portions of his tenth grade educational assessment indicated that Jared's overall reading skills including his reading comprehension abilities, and his math computation skills and knowledge, were very strong. He was presenting, however, academic delays in regard to many aspects of his applied math reasoning and math problem solving capabilities, as well as in regard to his organizational writing skills.

Based on the assessment findings from his updated tenth grade educational evaluation, which included a consideration of his past and recent academic difficulties, Jared was identified as having specific learning disabilities in mathematics and writing, with an emphasis on deficits involving organizational and sequential reasoning in multiple areas of higher-order mathematics and language arts. An Individualized Educational Plan was subsequently established for Jared which included weekly individual and small group remedial instructions in math and organizational writing. Some of the specific instructional areas in Jared's Individualized Educational Plan included:

Teaching Jared multiple organizational strategies and skills specifically focusing on the application of those teaching in math related contexts

Teaching Jared strategies for idea generation in math related contexts and activities

Progressively teaching Jared effective self-monitoring

and related executive learning and studying strategies specifically in relation to math related contexts and activities

Progressively teaching Jared multiple ways to analyze math questions and math word problems

Teaching Jared an extended core of math vocabularies and alternate ways of analyzing the language and forms of a math problem that would better allow him to understanding and solve mathematical questions

Providing Jared with multiple problem-solving templates to better provide him with step-by-step guidelines to follow once he identified what a particular the questions and nature of a given math problem

Providing Jared with individualized instructions focused on continuing improvement of his organizational writing skills. To that end, Jared was taught and allowed ample opportunities to practice how to develop and generate initial drafts of writing based on a primary general outline. He was additionally taught and encouraged to practice and use various techniques to allow him to "brainstorm" ideas and then systematically organize that written information into outlines and various forms of graphic representations. Jared was progressively taught and allowed to practice a range of sequential and organizational writing strategies that helped him to more effectively break down writing tasks and assignments into organized and manageable steps, and allowed for more systematic ways of developing and utilizing multiple and sequential edits when writing for organization of ideas, content, grammar, syntax, punctuation, and spelling. Consistent feedback was provided to Jared by his teachers on all of the new skills that he was taught, and were consistently reinforced in the contexts of his daily classroom work and his homework. Jared was also provided with individualized instructions and training in the applied knowledge and use of word processing programs, with a specific focus on learning and utilizing various writing tools common in word processing such as "cut and paste" and "spell check" functions.

NEURODEVELOPMENTAL FUNCTIONS AND MATH LEARNING DISORDERS

Attention Deficits

In math, students with attention regulation difficulties may:

- Have many careless math errors due to deficient self-monitoring (e.g., misreading plus and minus signs and other details in calculation
- Have difficulties initiating and continuing math assignments
- Have inconsistent levels of general output on math-related tasks
- Have poorly organized writing due to deficient self-monitoring
- Have mental fatigue, tiredness, and ultimate lack of persistence on math-related tasks
- Have inconsistent and uneven memory functions (Barkley, 1997, 1998; Dawson & Guare, 2004; Emerson & Babtie, 2010; Henderson, 2012; Levine, 1998, 2002a, 2002b; Lyon & Krasnegor, 2005; Pennington, 2009; Sousa, 2008)

Language Deficits

In learning math, students with language disabilities may have difficulties with math word problems as the language involved in such math processes may be experienced as convoluted, complex, and confusing (Dawson & Guare, 2004; Emerson & Babtie, 2010; Henderson, 2012; Levine, 1998, 2002a, 2002b; Lyon & Krasnegor, 2005; Pennington, 2009; Sousa, 2008).

Memory Deficits

In learning math, students with memory deficits may:

- Have difficulties with factual memory, required for rote math memory and math facts (for instance, memorizing times tables and basic math facts)
- Have poor recall of calculation rules for problem-solving activities
- Have an inconsistent flow of thinking (Berninger & Richards, 2002; Emerson & Babtie, 2010; Geary, 2013; Hale & Fiorello, 2004; Henderson, 2012; Lerew, 2005; Levine, 1998, 2002a, 2002b; Lyon & Krasnegor, 2005; Pennington, 2009)

Temporal-Sequential Ordering Deficits

In learning math, students with temporal-sequential ordering deficits may:

- Have difficulties with order and sequence processes within the context of various math-related activities (for instance, problems with correct order processes in division, multiplication, and fraction concepts)
- Have difficulty in number and letter formation
- Have transposed numbers and letters and data omissions
- Have poor sequencing processes
- Have developmentally poor problem-solving cohesiveness
- Have developmentally poor general organization and output (Levine, 1998, 2002a, 2002b; Lyon & Krasnegor, 2005)

Spatial Ordering Deficits

In learning math, students with spatial ordering deficits may:

- Have difficulties involving visual-spatial processing and mental imagery, which often play a very important role in conceptual and applied mathematics, such as understanding applied geometry principles
- Show uneven spacing between letters and words
- Use lines and margins ineffectively
- Have poor or disorganized spatial page planning
- Have general visual organization difficulties (Emerson & Babtie, 2010; Henderson, 2012; Levine, 1998, 2002a, 2002b)

Neuromotor Deficits

In learning math, students with neuromotor deficits, especially in the form of graphomotor delays, may:

- Have slow and laborious handwriting
- Have poor writing legibility
- Have an awkward or inefficient pencil grasp
- Have developmentally poor written fluency
- May write developmentally slowly and with great effort
- May find it hard to form numbers, symbols, and letters (Ball, 2002; Boon, 2010; Emerson & Babtie, 2010; Geary, 2013; Hale & Fiorello, 2004; Henderson, 2012; Jones, 2005; Kirby & Drew, 2003; Kurtz, 2007; Lerew, 2005; Levine, 1998, 2002a, 2002b; Lyon & Krasnegor, 2005; Ripley, 2001)

Higher-Order Cognition and Language Deficits

In learning math, students with higher-order cognition and language deficits may:

- Have difficulty developing, organizing, and expanding ideas
- Have difficulties with the understanding and development of abstract ideas
- Have difficulty with activities that require creativity and/or critical thinking

- Present developmentally simple and concrete ideas
- Typically only generate developmentally limited output when required (Emerson & Babtie, 2010; Geary, 2013; Hale & Fiorello, 2004; Henderson, 2012; Lerew, 2005; Levine, 1998, 2002a, 2002b; Lyon & Krasnegor, 2005)

Executive Function Deficits

In learning math, students with executive function deficits may:

- Have poor overall organizational skills
- Have poor idea generation
- Often develop poorly organized problem-solving sequences
- Often perseverate on a particular math rule or problem-solving strategy
- Often shift ideas poorly
- Have poor planning abilities in problem-solving construction and development
- Typically have poor self-monitoring and editing abilities
- Adequately initiate a math activity, but may have difficulty completing it (Barkley, 1997, 1998; Dawson & Guare, 2004; Emerson & Babtie, 2010; Henderson, 2012; Levine, 1998, 2002a, 2002b; Lyon & Krasnegor, 2005; Meltzer, 2007; Vargo et al., 2010; Yeager & Yeager, 2013)

Chapter 12

FINAL THOUGHTS

If I have seen further it is by standing on the shoulders of giants.

ISAAC NEWTON, 1675

A primary goal of this book is to provide practical and useful information to individuals interested in neurodevelopmental disorders. The book was developed and written with the goal of being a valuable learning tool and resource for educators, clinicians, medical professionals, parents, and all others who may be interested in obtaining initial or additional applied conceptual knowledge in the topic areas.

An important foundation of the book involves an in-depth exploration of neurodevelopmental constructs and related aspects of learning. Those constructs are specifically presented within the contexts of cognitive processes and functions that are typically compromised in the varying disorders of neurodevelopment. Each chapter includes a consistent continuation of the theme of cognitive constructs related to each area of neurodevelopmental functioning and disabilities, concurrent with clinical information pertinent to each specific disorder and diagnostic profile.

Another important function of this book is to provide a sound theoretical bridge for readers to make a direct connection between clinical and cognitive dimensions of the various neurodevelopmental disorders and learning problems and disabilities. As such, this book provides a unique understanding of various learning disabilities and related theories of learning based on integrated models of the contemporary neurosciences, cognitive psychology, neuropsychology, and applied educational psychology.

GLOBAL IMPLICATIONS

This book has presented various frameworks and definitions of learning disabilities. It has shown that while most definitions of specific learning disorders acknowledge the physiological etiologies of such learning dysfunctions, the legal definitions can vary widely across educational systems at regional, national, and even local levels. It is emphasized, however, that neurodevelopmental disorders can be characterized as impairments of the brain and central nervous system. More specifically, disorders of neurodevelopment (which include specific disabilities in language, reading, written language, and mathematics) are now widely accepted and consistently defined as conditions of abnormal brain function that adversely effect an individual's emotional and social functioning and cognitive and learning capabilities over time and across human developmental stages. From these perspectives, the phenomenon of learning disabilities and all other disorders of neurodevelopment transcend legal definitions and disagreements, as the ultimate physiological causes of all of these disorders and related cognitive dysfunctions make them common to the human experience. If so, then it follows that the information in this book is applicable and of value across boundaries of language, culture, and diverse educational systems and models.

ON THE SHOULDERS OF GIANTS

In 1675, the scientist Isaac Newton wrote, "If I have seen further it is by standing on the shoulders of giants." In that statement, this great man and pivotal historical figure acknowledged the previous scientists and all others before him who collectively developed a foundation of knowledge for him to expand on. This author is also both grateful for and humbled by those who came before and is deeply proud to be a small part of the process of the human quest for and acquisition of knowledge.

All empirical knowledge and information that develops over time is cumulative, and is continuously enhanced, modified, and expanded as new discoveries and information are acquired through established scientific methods. These processes of learning and understanding, in all of their elegance and beauty, are a crowning achievement of humankind. We can be assured, then, that as the various disciplines in the neurosciences, psychology, education, and other related professional and scientific fields provide us with new ongoing discoveries and data, our understandings of the neurodevelopmental disorders and related functions of learning will continuously be expanded, and all of us in the human family and our global society will benefit from those processes.

References

Adams, M. J. (1998). *Beginning to read: Thinking and learning about print.* Cambridge, MA: MIT Press.

Agaliotis, A. (2009). *Effective instructional interventions for students with learning disabilities in mathematics.* In G. D. Sideridis & T. A. Citro (Eds.), *Classroom strategies for struggling learners.* Weston, MA: Learning Disabilities Worldwide.

Akmajian, A., Demers, R., & Harnish, R. (1988). *Linguistics: An introduction to language and communication.* Cambridge, MA: MIT Press.

American Association on Intellectual and Developmental Disabilities (AAIDD). (2014). Retrieved from http://www.aaidd/intellectualdisabilities.com

American College of Obstetricians and Gynecologists. (2014). Fetal alcohol spectrum disorders. Retrieved from http://acog.org.

American Psychiatric Association. (2000). *Diagnostic and statistical manual of mental disorders* (4th ed., text rev.). Washington, DC: American Psychiatric Publishing.

American Psychiatric Association. (2013). *Diagnostic and statistical manual of mental disorders* (5th ed.). Arlington, VA: American Psychiatric Publishing.

American Speech-Language-Hearing Association. (1991). Learning disabilities: Issues on definition. Retrieved from http://www.asha.org/policy.

Aram, D. M., & Nation, J. E. (1980). Preschool language disorders and subsequent language and academic difficulties. *Journal of Communication Disorders, 13,* 159–170.

Armstrong, D. D. (2005). Neuropathology of Rett syndrome. *Journal of Child Neurology, 20,* 747–753.

Armstrong, K., Hangauer, J., & Nadeau, J. (2012). Use of intelligence tests in the identification of children with intellectual and developmental disabilities. In D. P. Flanagan & P. L. Harrison (Eds.), *Contemporary intellectual assessment: Theories, tests and issues*. New York: Guilford.

Arnstein, L., & Brown, R. (2005). Providing neuropsychological services to children exposed prenatally and perinatally to neurotoxins and deprivation. In R. D'Amato, E. Fletcher-Janzen, & C. Reynolds (Eds.), *Handbook of school neuropsychology*. Hoboken, NJ: Wiley.

Ashcraft, M. (1989). *Human memory and cognition*. Boston: Scott, Foresman.

Atwood, T. (1998). *Asperger's syndrome: A guide for parents and professionals*. London: Jessica Kingsley.

Atwood, T. (2008). An overview of autism spectrum disorders. In K. D. Buron & P. Wolfberg (Eds.), *Learners on the autism spectrum: Preparing highly qualified educators*. Shawnee Mission, KS: Autism Asperger.

Ayers, A. J. (1972). *Sensory integration and learning disorders*. Los Angeles: Western Psychological Services.

Baddeley, A. (2000). Working memory: The interface between memory and cognition. In M. S. Gazzaniga (Ed.), *Cognitive neuroscience: A reader*. Oxford, UK: Blackwell.

Baddeley, A. (2013). *Essentials of human memory*. New York: Taylor and Francis.

Baker, L., & Cantwell, D. P. (1987). Comparison of well, emotionally disturbed, and behaviorally disordered children with linguistic problems. *Journal of the American Academy of Child and Adolescent Psychiatry, 26*, 193–196.

Ball, M. (2002). *Developmental coordination disorder*. New York: Routledge.

Barkley, R. A. (1997). *ADHD and the nature of self-control*. New York: Guilford.

Barkley, R. A. (1998). *Attention deficit hyperactivity disorder: A handbook for diagnosis and treatment* (2nd ed.). New York: Guilford.

Barnes, M., Fuchs, L., & Ewing-Cobbs, L. (2010). Math disabilities. In K. Yeates, M. Ris, H. Taylor, & B. Pennington (Eds.), *Pediatric neuropsychology: Research, theory, and practice*. New York: Guilford.

Baron, I., Fennel, E., & Voeller, K. (1995). *Pediatric neuropsychology in the medical setting*. Oxford, UK: Oxford University Press.

Barry, S., Baird, G., Lascelles, K., Bunton, P., & Hedderly, T. (2011). Neurodevelopmental movement disorders: An update on childhood motor stereotypes. *Developmental Medicine and Child Neurology, 53*(11), 979–985.

Bartlett, F. C. (1932). *Remembering*. Cambridge, UK: Cambridge University Press.

Batchelor, E., & Dean, R. (Eds.) (1996). *Pediatric neuropsychology: Interfacing assessment and treatment for rehabilitation*. Boston: Allyn and Bacon.

Batshaw, M. (1997). *Children with disabilities* (4th ed.). Baltimore, MD: Paul H. Brookes.

Baty, B., Carey, J., & McMahon, W. (2011). Neurodevelopmental disorders and medical genetics: An overview. In S. Goldstein & C. Reynolds (Eds.), *Handbook of neurodevelopmental and genetic disorders in children* (2nd ed.). New York: Guilford.

Bauman, M., & Kemper, T. (1994). *The neurobiology of autism.* Baltimore, MD: Johns Hopkins University Press.

Baumberger, J. P., & Harper, R. E. (1999). *Assisting students with disabilities: What school counselors can and must do.* Thousand Oaks, CA: Corwin.

Bauminger-Zviely, N. (2013). *Social and academic abilities in children with high functioning autism spectrum disorders.* New York: Guilford.

Beamon, G. W. (1997). *Sparking the thinking of students, ages 10–14: Strategies for teachers.* Thousand Oaks, CA: Corwin.

Beamon, G. W. (2001). *Teaching with adolescent learning in mind.* Thousand Oaks, CA: Corwin.

Benasich, A. A. (2012). Potential early precursors of specific language impairment and dyslexia. In A. A. Benasich & R. H. Fitch (Eds.), *Developmental dyslexia: Early precursors, neurobehavioral markers, and biological substrates.* Baltimore, MD: Paul H. Brookes.

Benasich, A. A., & Fitch, R. H. (2012). *Developmental dyslexia: Early precursors, neurobehavioral markers, and biological substrates.* Baltimore, MD: Paul H. Brookes.

Benjafield, J. G. (2005). *A history of psychology* (2nd ed.). Don Mills, ON: Oxford University Press.

Berninger, V. W. (2008). Defining and differentiating dysgraphia, dyslexia, and language learning disability within a working memory model. In M. Mody & E. R. Silliman (Eds.), *Brain, behavior, and learning in language and reading disorders.* New York: Guilford.

Berninger, V. (2010). Assessing and intervening with children with written language disorders. In D. Miller (Ed.), *Best practices in school neuropsychology: Guidelines for effective practice, assessment, and evidence-based intervention.* Hoboken, NJ: Wiley.

Berninger, V., & Richards, T. (2002). *Brain literacy for educators and psychologists.* Boston: Academic.

Berninger, V. W., & Wolf, B. J. (2009). *Teaching students with dyslexia and dysgraphia: Lessons from teaching and science.* Baltimore: Paul H. Brooks.

Bivina, L., Moghaddam, B., & Wardinsky, T. D. (2013). Down syndrome. In R. Hanson & S. Rogers (Eds.), *Autism and other neurodevelopmental disorders. Arlington, VA: American Psychiatric Publishing.*

Blachman, B. (1997). *Foundations of reading acquisition and dyslexia: Implications for early intervention.* Mahwah, NJ: Lawrence Erlbaum.

Boa, X., Downs, J., Wong, K., Williams, S., & Leonard, H. (2013). Using a large international sample to investigate epilepsy in Rett syndrome. *Developmental Medicine and Child Neurology, 55*(6), 553–558.

Bolton, P. F., Carcani-Rathwell, I., Hutton, J., Goode, S., Howlin, P., & Rutter, M. (2011). Features and correlates of epilepsy in autism. *British Journal of Psychiatry, 198*, 289–294.

Boon, M. (2010). *Understanding dyspraxia*. Philadelphia: Jessica Kingsley.

Borkowski, J. G. (1985). Signs of intelligence: Strategy generalization and metacognition. In S. R. Yussen (Ed.), *The growth of reflection in children* (pp. 105–144). Orlando, FL: Academic Press.

Borod, J. (Ed.) (2000). *The neuropsychology of emotion*. New York: Oxford University Press.

Bradley, L., & Bryant, P. E. (1983). Categorizing sounds and learning to read: A causal connection. *Nature, 301*, 419–421.

Brady, S., Shankweiler, D., & Mann, V. (1983). Speech perception and memory coding in relation to reading ability. *Journal of Experimental Child Psychology, 35*, 345–367.

Breier, J. I., Simos, P. J., Fletcher, J. M., Castillo, E. M., Zhang, W., & Papanicolaou, A. C. (2003). Abnormal activation of temporoparietal language areas during phonetic analysis in children with dyslexia. *Neuropsychology, 17*, 610–621.

Bronson, M. B. (2000). *Self-regulation in early childhood*. New York: Guilford.

Brown, R. T., & McMillan, K. M. (2011). Rett syndrome: A truly pervasive developmental disorder. In S. Goldstein & C. Reynolds (Eds.), *Handbook of neurodevelopmental and genetic disorders in children (2nd ed.)*. New York: Guilford.

Brown, R. T., McMillan, K. K., & Herschthal, A. (2005). Rett syndrome. In S. Goldstein & C. R. Reynolds (Eds.), *Handbook of neurodevelopmental and genetic disorders in adults* (pp. 383–409). New York: Guilford.

Buron, K. D., & Wolfberg, P. (Eds.) (2008). *Learners on the autism spectrum: Preparing highly qualified educators*. Shawnee Mission, KS: Autism Asperger.

Bursuck, W., & Dickson, S. (1999). Implementing a model for preventing reading failure: A report from the field. *Learning Disabilities Research and Practice, 14*(4), 191–202.

Byrnes, J. (2001). *Minds, brains, and learning: Understanding the psychological and educational relevance of neuroscientific research*. New York: Guilford.

Camarata, S., Hughes, C., & Ruhl, K. (1988). Mild/moderate behaviorally disordered students: A population at risk for language disorders. *Language, Speech, and Hearing Services in Schools, 19*, 191–200.

Campione, J. C., & Brown, A. L. (1978). Toward a theory of intelligence: Contributions from research with retarded children. *Intelligence, 2*, 279–304.

Cantwell, D. P., & Baker, L. (1977). Psychiatric disorders in children with speech and language retardation: A clinical review. *Archives of General Psychiatry, 34,* 583–591.

Carroll, J. B. (1997). The three-stratum theory of cognitive abilities. In D. P. Flanagan, J. L. Genshaft, & P. L. Harrison (Eds.), *Contemporary intellectual assessment: Theories, tests, and issues* (pp. 122–130). New York: Guilford.

Carter, R. (2009). *The human brain book.* London: DK.

Castellanos, F. X., Lee, P. P., Sharp, W., Jeffries, N. O., Greenstein, D. K., & Clasen, L. S. (2002). Developmental trajectories of brain volume abnormalities in children with attention deficit/hyperactivity disorder. *Journal of the American Medical Association, 288,* 1740–1748.

Cattell, R. B. (1943). The measurement of adult intelligence. *Psychological Bulletin, 40,* 153–193.

Cattell, R. B. (1963). Theory of fluid and crystallized intelligence: A critical experiment. *Journal of Educational Psychology, 54,* 1–22.

Cattell, R. B., & Horn, J. L. (1978). A check on the theory of fluid and crystallized intelligence with descriptions of new subtest designs. *Journal of Educational Measurement, 15*(3), 139–164.

Catts, H. W. (1996). Defining dyslexia as a language disorder: An expanded view. *Topics in Language Disorders, 16*(2), 14–29.

Catts, H., & Kamhi, A. (1999). *Language and reading disabilities.* Boston: Allyn and Bacon.

Cavanna, A. E. & Seri, S. (2013). Tourette's syndrome. *British Medical Journal, 347,* 26–30.

Cazden, C. B. (1986). Classroom discourse. In M. C. Wittrock (Ed.), *Handbook of research on teaching* (pp. 432–464). New York: Macmillan.

Chambers, M. E., Sugden, D. A., & Sinani, C. (2005). The nature of children with developmental coordination disorder. In D. Sugden & M. Chambers (Eds.), *Children with developmental coordination disorder.* London: Whurr.

Chaste, P., Betancur, C., Gerard-Blanluet, M., Bargiacchi, B., Kuzbari, S., Drunat, S., Leboyer, M., Bourgeron, T., & Delorme, R. (2012). High functioning autism spectrum disorder and fragile X syndrome: Report of two affected sisters. *Molecular Autism, 3(1),* 5–10.

Chittooran, M., & Tait, R. (2005). Understanding and Implementing neuropsychologically based written language interventions. In R. D'Amato, E. Fletcher-Janzen, & C. Reynolds (Eds.), *Handbook of school neuropsychology.* Hoboken, NJ: Wiley.

Cicchetti, D., & Beeghly, M. (1990). *Down syndrome: A developmental perspective.* Cambridge: Cambridge University Press.

Cimera, R. E. (2007). *Learning disabilities: What are they?* Lanham, MD: Rowman and Littlefield Education.

Cocchi, G., Gualdi, S., Bower, C., Halliday, J., Jonsson, B., Myrelid, A., et al. (2010). International trends of Down syndrome 1993–2004: Births in relation to maternal age and terminations of pregnancies. *Birth Defects Research, Part A, 88,* 747–749.

Cohen, G., Eysenck, M., & LeVoi, M. (1986). *Memory: A cognitive approach.* Milton Keynes, UK: Open University Press.

Cohen, N., Davine, M., & Meloche-Kelly, M. (1989). Prevalence of unsuspected language disorders in a child psychiatric population. *Journal of the American Academy of Child and Adolescent Psychiatry, 28,* 107–111.

Coles, R. (1970). *Erik Erikson: The growth of his work.* Boston: Little, Brown.

Cook, E. H., & Leventhal, B. L. (1992). Neuropsychiatric disorders of childhood and adolescence. In S. C. Yudofsky & R. E. Hales (Eds.), *The American Psychiatric Press textbook of neuropsychiatry* (2nd ed.). Washington, DC: American Psychiatric Press.

Corbett, B., & Gunther, J. (2011). Autism spectrum disorders. In S. Goldstein & C. Reynolds (Eds.), *Handbook of neurodevelopmental and genetic disorders in children (2nd Ed.). New York: Guilford.*

Corbett, B., & Schulte, T. (2011). Autism spectrum disorders. In *Handbook of neurodevelopmental and genetic disorders in children* (2nd ed.). New York: Guilford.

Corey, G. (2005). *Theory and practice of counseling and psychotherapy* (7th ed.). Belmont, CA: Wadsworth.

Cornish, K., Turk, J., & Hagerman, R. (2008). The fragile X continuum: New advances and perspectives. *Journal of Intellectual Disability Research, 52(6),* 469–482.

Corsini, R. J., & Wedding, D. (Eds.) (2004). *Current psychotherapies* (7th ed.). Belmont, CA: Wadsworth.

Council for Exceptional Children. (2014). Who are exceptional learners. Retrieved from http://www.cec.sped.org/special-ed-topics/Who-Are-Exceptional-Learners?

Cozolino, L. (2006). *The neuroscience of human relationships.* New York: Norton.

Crawford, G. (2007). *Brain-based teaching with adolescent learning in mind.* Thousand Oaks, CA: Corwin.

Daly, E. J., Chafouleas, S., & Skinner, C. H. (2005). *Interventions for reading problems: Designing and evaluating effective strategies.* New York: Guilford.

D'Amato, R., Fletcher-Janzen, E., & Reynolds, C. (Eds.) (2005). *Handbook of school neuropsychology.* Hoboken, NJ: Wiley.

Dass, J. P., Naglieri, J. A., & Kirby, J. R. (1994). *Assessment of cognitive processes: The PASS theory of intelligence.* Needham Heights, MA: Allyn and Bacon.

Dawson, P. (2010). Lazy—or not? *Educational Leadership, 68(2),* 35–38.

Dawson, P., & Guare, R. (2004). *Executive skills in children and adolescents: A practical guide to assessment and intervention.* New York: Guilford.

Decker, S., & Davis, A. (2010). Assessing and intervening with children with sensory-motor impairment. In D. Miller (Ed.), *Best practices in school neuropsychology: Guidelines for effective practice, assessment, and evidence-based intervention.* Hoboken, NJ: Wiley.

Denckla, M. B. (1972). Color-naming deficits in dyslexic boys. *Cortex, 8,* 164–176.

Denckla, M. B., Barquero, L. A., Lindstrom, E. R., Benedict, S. L., Wilson, L. M., & Cutting, L. E. (2013). Attention deficit/hyperactivity disorder, executive function, and reading comprehension: Different but related. In H. L. Swanson, K. R. Harris, & S. Graham (Eds.), *Handbook of learning disabilities* (2nd ed.). New York: Guilford.

Denckla, M. B., & Rudel, R. G. (1974). "Rapid automatized naming" of pictured objects, colors, letters, and numbers by normal children. *Brain and Language, 3,* 1–15.

DeOrnellas, K., Hood, J., & Novales, B. (2010). Assessing and intervening with children with Asperger's disorder. In D. Miller (Ed.), *Best practices in school neuropsychology: Guidelines for effective practice, assessment, and evidence-based intervention.* Hoboken, NJ: Wiley.

De Vries, L. B. A., Halley, D. J. J., Oostra, B. A., & Niermeijer, M. F. (1994). The fragile-X syndrome: A growing gene causing familial intellectual disability. Journal of Intellectual Disability Research, 38(1), 1–8.

Donald, A. G., & Shah, N. S. (Eds.) (2013). *Movement disorders.* New York: Springer.

Dooley, C. (2010). Assessing and intervening with children with developmental delays. In D. Miller (Ed.), *Best practices in school neuropsychology: Guidelines for effective practice, assessment, and evidence-based intervention.* Hoboken, NJ: Wiley.

Drew, S., & Creek, J. (2005). *Developmental coordination disorders in adults.* Hoboken, NJ: Wiley.

Drozdick, L. W., Wahlstrom, D., Zhu, J., & Weiss, L. G. (2012). The Wechsler Adult Intelligence Scale—Fourth Edition and the Wechsler Memory Scale—Fourth Edition. In D. P. Flanagan & P. L. Harrison (Eds.), *Contemporary intellectual assessment: Theories, tests and issues.* New York: Guilford.

Dudley-Marling, C., & Searle, D. (1988). Enriching language learning environments for students with learning disabilities. *Journal of Learning Disabilities, 21,* 140–143.

Duke, N. K., Cartwright, K. B., & Hilden, K. R. (2014). Difficulties with reading comprehension. In C. A. Stone, E. R. Silliman, B. J. Ehren, & G. P. Wallach (Eds.), *Handbook of language and literacy: Development and disorders.* New York: Guilford.

Durand, V. M. (2013). Sleep problems in autism spectrum disorder: Assessment and treatment. In J. K. Luiselli (Ed.), *Children and youth with autism spectrum disorder(ASD): Recent advances and innovations in assessment, education, and intervention.* New York: Oxford University Press.

Durand, V. M. (2014). *Autism spectrum disorder: A clinical guide for general practitioners.* Washington, DC: American Psychological Association.

Durston, S. (2003). A review of the biological basis of ADHD: What have we learned from imaging studies? *Mental Retardation and Developmental Disabilities Research Reviews, 9,* 184–195.

Duska, R., & Whelan, M. (1975). *Moral development: A guide to Piaget and Kohlburg.* Mahwah, NJ: Paulist Press.

Dykens, E. M., & Lense, M. (2011). Intellectual disabilities and autism spectrum disorder: A cautionary note. In D. G. Amaral, G. Dawson, & D. Geschwind (Eds.), *Autism spectrum disorders.* New York: Oxford University Press.

Emerson, J., & Babtie, P. (2010). *The dyscalculia assessment.* London: Continuum.

Erikson, E. (1993). *Childhood and society.* New York:Norton.

Escalante-Mead, R., Minshew, N., & Sweeney, J. (2003). Abnormal brain lateralization in high-functioning autism. *Journal of Autism and Developmental Disorders, 33,* 539–544.

Fadiman, J., & Frager, R. (2002). *Personality and personal growth* (5th ed.). Upper Saddle River, NJ: Prentice Hall.

Fang, Z., Schleppegrell, M. J., & Moore, J. (2014). The linguistic challenges of learning across academic disciplines. In C. A. Stone, E. R. Silliman, B. J. Ehren, & G. P. Wallach (Eds.), *Handbook of language and literacy: Development and disorders.* New York: Guilford.

Farran, E., & Karmiloff-Smith, A. (2012). *Neurodevelopmental disorders across the lifespan: A neuroconstructivist approach.* New York: Oxford University Press.

Fawcett, A., & Nicolson, R. (2001). Speed and temporal processing in dyslexia. In M. Wolf (Ed.), *Dyslexia, fluency, and the brain.* Timonium, MD: York Press.

Feifer, S. (2010). Assessing and intervening with children with reading disorders. In D. Miller (Ed.), *Best practices in school neuropsychology: Guidelines for effective practice, assessment, and evidence-based intervention.* Hoboken, NJ: Wiley.

Feifer, S., & DeFina, P. (2000). *The neuropsychology of reading disorders: Diagnosis and intervention workbook.* Middletown, MD: School Neuropsych Press.

Feifer, S., & DeFina, P. (2002). *The neuropsychology of written language disorders.* Middletown, MD: School Neuropsych Press.

Feifer, S. G., & Della Toffalo, D. A. (2007). Integrating RTI with cognitive psychology: A scientific approach to reading. Middletown, MD: School Neuropsych Press.

Flanagan, D. P., Genshaft, J. L., & Harrison, P. L. (1997). *Contemporary intellectual assessment: Theories, tests, and issues.* New York: Guilford.

Flanagan, D. P., & Harrison, P. L. (Eds.) (2012). *Contemporary intellectual assessment: Theories, tests and issues* (3rd ed.). New York: Guilford.

Fletcher, G., Lyon, G., Fuchs, L., & Barnes, M. (2007). *Learning disabilities: From identification to intervention*. New York: Guilford.

Fletcher, J. M. (1996). Executive functions in children: Introduction to the special series. *Developmental Neuropsychology, 12*, 1–3.

Fletcher, J. M., Stuebing, K. K., Morris, R. D., & Lyon, G. R. (2013). Classification and definition of learning disabilities: A hybrid model. In H. L. Swanson, K. R. Harris, & S. Graham (Eds.), *Handbook of learning disabilities* (2nd ed.). New York: Guilford.

Foundation for People With Learning Disabilities. (2014). Definition of learning disabilities. Retrieved from http://www.learningdisabilities. org.uk/about-learning-disabilities/definition-learning disabilities.

Freeman, R. D., & Soltanifar, A. (2010). Stereotypic movement disorder: Easily missed. *Developmental Medicine and Child Neurology, 52*(8), 733–738.

Freitag, C. M., Kleser, C., Schneider, M., & von Gontard, A. (2007). Quantitative Assessment of Neuromotor Function in Adolescents of High Functioning Autism and Asperger Syndrome. *Journal of Autism and Developmental Disorders, 37*(5), 948–959.

Frith, U. (2008). *Autism: A very short introduction*. New York: Oxford University Press.

Gallahue, D. (1992). *Understanding motor development in children*. London: Wiley.

Gardner, H. (1983). *Frames of mind: The theory of multiple intelligences*. New York: Basic Books.

Garnett, K. (1998). Math learning disabilities. *Division for Learning Disabilities Journal of the Council for Exceptional Children*.

Garralda, M., & Raynaud, J. (2012). *Brain, mind, and developmental psychopathology in childhood*. New York: Jason Aronson.

Gazzaniga, M. S. (2000). *Cognitive neuroscience: A reader*. Oxford, UK: Blackwell.

Geary, D. (1993). Mathematical disabilities: Cognitive, neuropsychological, and genetic components. *Psychological Bulletin, 114*, 345–362.

Geary, D. (2000). Mathematical disorders: An overview for educators. *Perspectives, 26*(3), 6–9.

Geary, D. (2013). Learning disabilities in mathematics: Recent advances. In H. L. Swanson, K. R. Harris, & S. Graham (Eds.), *Handbook of learning disabilities* (2nd ed.). New York: Guilford

Geschwind, N. (1965). Disconnection syndrome in animals and man (parts I, II). *Brain, 88*, 237–294, 585–644.

Geuze, R. H. (2005). Cognitive explanations of the planning and organization of music. In D. Sugden & M. Chambers (Eds.), *Children with developmental coordination disorder*. London: Whurr.

Ghaziuddin, M. (2005). *Mental health aspects of autism and Asperger syndrome*. London: Jessica Kingsley.

Ghaziuddin, M., Ghaziuddin, N., & Gredden, J. (2002). Depression in persons with autism: Implications for research and clinical care. *Research in Autism Spectrum Disorders, 32,* 299–306.

Ginsburg, H., & Opper, S. (1987). *Piaget's theory of intellectual development* (3rd ed.). Upper Saddle River, NJ: Prentice Hall.

Goodman, K. S. (1976). Reading: A psycholinguistic guessing game. In H. Singer & R. Ruddell (Eds.), *Theoretical models and processing of reading* (pp. 497–501). Newark, DE: International Reading Association.

Goodman, K. S., Bird, L. B., & Goodman, Y. M. (1992). *The whole language catalogue: Supplement on authentic assessment.* New York: SRA Macmillan.

Goodman, K., & Goodman, Y. (1982). A whole language comprehension centered view of reading development. In L. Reed & S. Ward (Eds.), *Basic skills: Issues and choices* (pp. 125–134). St. Louis, MO: CEMREL.

Goldberg, E. (2001). *The executive brain: Frontal lobes and the civilized mind.* New York: Oxford University Press.

Goldstein, S. (2011). Attention deficit/hyperactivity disorder. In S. Goldstein & C. Renolds (Eds.), *Handbook of neurodevelopmental and genetic disorders in children* (2nd ed.). New York: Guilford.

Goldstein, S., & Reynolds, C. (2011). *Handbook of neurodevelopmental and genetic disorders in children* (2nd ed.). New York: Guilford.

Goswami, U. (2008). *Cognitive development: The learning brain.* New York: Taylor and Francis.

Greene, J., & Coulson, M. (1995). *Language understanding: Current issues* (2nd ed.). Buckingham, PA: Open University Press.

Groth-Marnat, G. (Ed.) (2000). *Neuropsychological assessment in clinical practice: A guide to test interpretation and integration.* New York: Wiley.

Gruber, H., & Voneche, J. (Eds.) (1995). *The essential Piaget: An interpretative reference and guide.* New York: Jason Aronson.

Gualtieri, C. T., Koriath, U., Bourgondien, M., & Saleeby, N. (1983). Language disorders in children referred for psychiatric services. *Journal of the American Academy of Child Psychiatry, 22,* 165–171.

Hagberg, B. (1995). Rett syndrome: Clinical peculiarities and biological mysteries. *Acta Paediatrica, 84,* 971–976.

Hagerman, R. J. (2011). Fragile X syndrome and fragile X-associated disorders. In S. Goldstein & C. Reynolds (Eds.), *Handbook of neurodevelopmental and genetic disorders in children (2nd ed.). New York: Guilford.*

Halbach, N. S., Smeets, E. E., Steinbusch, C., Maaskant, M. A., Van Waardenburg, D., & Curfs, L. M. (2013). Aging in Rett syndrome: A longitudinal study. *Clinical Genetics, 84*(3), 223–229.

Hale, J., & Fiorello, C. (2004). *School psychology: A practicioner's handbook.* New York: Guilford.

Hale, J., Reddy, L., Wilcox, G., McLaughlin, A., Hain, L., Stern, A., Henzel, J., & Eusebio, E. (2010). Assessment and intervention practices for children with ADHD and other frontal-striatal circuit disorders. In D. Miller (Ed.), *Best practices in school neuropsychology: Guidelines for effective practice, assessment, and evidence-based intervention.* Hoboken, NJ: Wiley.

Hallahan, D. P., Pullen, P. C., & Ward, D. (2013). A brief history of the field of learning disabilities. In H. L. Swanson, K. R. Harris, & S. Graham (Eds.), *Handbook of learning disabilities* (2nd ed.). New York: Guilford.

Hallowell, E. M., & Ratey, J. J. (1994). *Driven to distraction: Recognizing and coping with attention deficit disorder from childhood through adulthood.* New York: Pantheon.

Hanks, S. (1990). Motor disabilities in the Rett syndrome and physical therapy strategies. *Brain and Development, 12,* 157–161.

Hanson, R., & Rogers, S. (Eds.) (2012). *Autism and other neurodevelopmental disorders.* Arlington, VA: American Psychiatric Publishing.

Hassiotis, A., Barron, D. A., & Hall, I. (2010). *Intellectual disability psychiatry: A practical handbook.* Hoboken, NJ: Wiley.

Hazlett, H. C., Hammer, J., Hooper, S. R., & Kamphaus, R. W. (2011). Down syndrome. In S. Goldstein & C. Reynolds (Eds.), *Handbook of neurodevelopmental and genetic disorders in children (2nd ed.).* New York: Guilford.

Hellend, T., & Asbjoernsen, A. (2000). Executive functions in dyslexia. *Child Neuropsychology, 6,* 37–48.

Henderson, A. (2012). *Dyslexia, dyscalculia and mathematics: A practical guide* (2nd ed.). New York: Routledge.

Hergenhahn, B. R. (2009). *An introduction to the history of psychology.* Belmont, CA: Wadsworth.

Hobsen, P. R. (2012). Autism, literal language and concrete thinking: Some developmental considerations. *Metaphor and Symbol, 27*(1), 4–21.

Hodapp, R., & Dykens, E. (2004). Intellectual disabilities: Definitions and classifications. In J. A. Rondal, R. M. Hodapp, S. Soresi, E. M. Dykens, & L. Nota (Eds.), *Intellectual disabilities: Genetics, behavior and inclusion.* London: Whurr.

Hodapp, R., & Dykens, E. (2012). Genetic disorders of intellectual disability: Expanding our concepts of phenotypes and family outcomes. Journal of Genetic Counseling, 6, 761–769.

Horn, J. L. (1968). Organization of abilities and the development of intelligence. *Psychological Review, 75,* 242–259.

Horn, J. L. (1979). Trends in the measurement of intelligence. *Intelligence, 3,* 229–239.

Horn, J. L. (1985). Remodeling old models of intelligence. In B. Wolman (Ed.), *Handbook of intelligence* (pp. 267–300). New York: Wiley.

Horn, J. L., & Noll, J. (1997). Human cognitive capabilities: Gf-Gc theory. In D. P. Flanagan, J. L. Genshaft, & P. L. Harrison (Eds.), *Contemporary intellectual assessment: Theories, tests, and issues* (pp. 53–91). New York: Guilford.

Houston, J. P. (1986). *Fundamentals of learning and memory* (3rd ed.). New York: Harcourt Brace Jovanovich.

Humphries, T., Koltun, H., Malone, M., & Roberts, W. (1994). Teacher-identified oral language difficulties among boys with attention problems. *Developmental and Behavioral Pediatrics, 15*, 92–98.

Hunter, K. (2007). *Rett syndrome handbook* (2nd ed.). Cincinnati, OH: International Rett Syndrome Foundation.

Hynd, G., & Cohen, M. (1983). *Dyslexia: Neuropsychological theory, research, and clinical differentiation.* Boston: Allyn and Bacon.

International Rett Syndrome Foundation (IRSF) (2008). About Rett syndrome. Retrieved from www.rett syndrome.org/About-Rett-Syndrome

Ivarsson, T., & Melin, K. (2008). Autism spectrum traits in children and adolescents with obsessive-compulsive disorder (OCD). *Journal of Anxiety Disorders, 22*, 969–978.

Jensen, A. R. (1993). Spearman's *g*: Links between psychometrics and biology. *Annals of the New York Academy of Sciences, 702*, 103–129.

Jensen, A. R. (1998). *The g factor: The science of mental ability.* Westport, CT: Praeger.

Jitendra, A. K., & Gajria, M. (2011). Main idea and summarization instruction to improve reading comprehension. In R. E. O'Connor & P. F. Vadasy (Eds.), *Handbook of reading interventions.* New York: Guilford.

Johnson, A. (2008). *Teaching reading and writing: A guidebook for tutoring and remediating students.* New York: Rowman and Littlefield Education.

Jones, N. (Ed.) (2005). *Developing school provision for children with dyspraxia: A practical guide.* Thousand Oaks, CA: Sage.

Jongmans, M. J. (2005). Assessment of handwriting in children with developmental coordination disorder. In D. Sugden & M. Chambers (Eds.), *Children with developmental coordination disorder.* London: Whurr.

Kahana, M. J. (2012). *Foundations of human memory.* New York: Oxford University Press.

Kahmi, A., & Catts, H. (1989). *Reading disabilities: A developmental language perspective.* Boston: Little, Brown.

Kahney, H. (1986). *Problem solving: A cognitive approach.* Philadelphia: Open University Press.

Kalat, J. (2004). *Biological psychology* (8th ed.). Toronto: Wadsworth.

Kame'enui, E., Simmons, D., Good, R., & Harn, B. (2001). The use of fluency-based measures in early identification and evaluation of intervention efficacy in schools. In M. Wolf (Ed.), *Dyslexia, fluency and the brain.* Timonium, MD: York Press.

Kamhi, A., & Catts, H. (1989). *Reading disabilities: A developmental language perspective.* Boston: Little, Brown.

Kandel, E. R., Schwartz, J. H., & Jessell, T. M. (2000). *Principles of neural science* (4th ed.). New York: McGraw-Hill.

Keenan, J. M. (2014). Assessment of reading comprehension. In C. A.

Stone, E. R. Silliman, B. J. Ehren, & G. P. Wallach (Eds.), *Handbook of language and literacy: Development and disorders.* New York: Guilford.

Kellogg, R. (2007). *Fundamentals of cognitive psychology.* Thousand Oaks, CA: Sage.

Kerns, K. A., Don, A., Mateer, C. A., & Streissguth, A. P. (1997). Cognitive deficits in nonretarded adults with fetal alcohol syndrome. *Journal of Learning Disabilities,* **30(6), 684–693.**

Kibby, M. Y. (2009). There are multiple contributors to the verbal short-term memory deficit in children with developmental reading disabilities. *Child Neuropsychology, 15*(5),485–506.

King, R., Jones, D., & Laskey, E. (1982). In retrospect: A fifteen year follow-up of speech and language-disordered children. *Language, Speech, and Hearing Services in Schools, 13,* 24–32.

Kirby, A., & Drew, S. (2003). *Guide to dyspraxia and developmental coordination disorders.* New York: Taylor and Francis.

Klein, R., & McMullen, P. (1999). *Converging methods for understanding reading and dyslexia.* Cambridge, MA: MIT Press.

Klingner, J. K., Morrison, A., & Eppolito, A. (2011). Metacognition to improve reading comprehension. In R. E. O'Connor & P. F. Vadasy (Eds.), *Handbook of reading interventions.* New York: Guilford.

Klingner, J., Vaughn, S., & Boardman, A. (2007). *Teaching reading comprehension to students with learning difficulties.* New York: Guilford.

Kolb, B., & Wishaw, I. (1990). *Fundamentals of neuropsychology* (3rd ed.). New York: Freeman.

Kolb, B., & Wishaw, I. (2009). *An introduction to brain and behavior* (3rd ed.). New York: Worth.

Kozey, M., & Siegel, L. S. (2008). Definition of learning disabilities in Canadian provinces and territories. *Canadian Psychology, 49*(2), 162–171.

Kuder, S. (2003). *Teaching students with language and communication disabilities.* Boston: Allyn and Bacon.

Kurtz, L. A. (2007). *Understanding motor skills in children with dyspraxia, ADHD, and other learning disabilities: A guide to improving coordination.* Philadelphia: Jessica Kingsley.

Lane, R. D., & Nadel, L. (Eds.) (2000). *Cognitive neuroscience of emotion.* New York: Oxford University Press.

Lang, M. (2010). Assessing and intervening with children with autism spectrum disorders. In D. Miller (Ed.), *Best practices in school neuropsychology: Guidelines for effective practice, assessment, and evidence-based intervention.* Hoboken, NJ: Wiley.

Learning Disabilities Association of America. (2014). Defining learning disabilities. Retrieved from http://www.ldaamerica.org/defining/learningdisabilities.

Learning Disabilities Association of Canada. (2014). Learning disabilities defined. Retrieved from http://www.ldac-acta.ca/learnmore/ld-defined.

Lebowitz, E. (2012). Tourette syndrome in youth with and without obsessive compulsive disorder and attention deficit hyperactivity disorder. *European Child and Adolescent Psychiatry, 21*(8), 451–457.

Ledford, J. R., & Gast, D. L. (2006). Feeding problems in children with autism spectrum disorder: A review. *Focus on Autism and Other Developmental Disabilities, 21,* 153–166.

Leigh, M. J. S., Hagerman, R. J., & Hessl, D. (2013). Fragile X syndrome. In R. Hanson & S. Rogers (Eds.), Autism and other neurodevelopmental disorders. Arlington, VA: American Psychiatric Publishing.

Lerew, C. (2005). Understanding and implementing neuropsychologically based arithmetic interventions. In R. D'Amato, E. Fletcher-Janzen, & C. Reynolds (Eds.), *Handbook of school neuropsychology.* Hoboken, NJ: Wiley.

Levine, M. (1995). Childhood neurodevelopmental dysfunction and learning disorders. *Harvard Mental Health Letter, 12*(1), 5.

Levine, M. (1998). *Developmental variation and learning disorders* (2nd ed.). Cambridge, MA: Educators Publishing Service.

Levine, M. (2002a). *Educational care: A system for understanding and helping children with learning problems at home and in school* (2nd ed.). Cambridge, MA: Educators Publishing Service.

Levine, M. (2002b). *A mind at a time.* New York: Simon and Schuster.

Lezak, M. D., Howieson, D. B., & Loring, D. W. (2004). *Neuropsychological assessment* (4th ed.). New York: Oxford University Press.

Lieberman, D. A. (2011). *Human learning and memory.* Cambridge: Cambridge University Press.

Love, A. J., & Thompson, M. G. (1988). Language disorders and attention deficit disorders in young children referred for psychiatric services. *American Journal of Orthopsychiatry, 58,* 52–63.

Luria, A. R. (1966a). *Higher cortical functions in man.* New York: Basic Books.

Luria, A. R. (1966b). *Human brain and psychological processes.* New York: Harper and Row.

Lyon, G. R. (1996). Learning disabilities. *Future of Children: Special Education for Students with Learning Disabilities, 6*(1), 54–73.

Lyon, G. R., & Krasnegor, N. A. (2005). *Attention, memory, and executive function.* Baltimore, MD: Paul H. Brookes.

Lyons, C. A. (2003). *Teaching struggling readers: How to use brain-based research to maximize learning.* Portsmouth, NH: Heinemann.

Mack, A., & Warr-Leeper, G. (1992). Language abilities in boys with chronic behavior disorders. *Language, Speech, and Hearing Services in Schools, 23,* 214–223.

Manis, F., Doi, L., & Bhada, B. (2000). Naming speed, phonological awareness, and orthographic knowledge in second graders. *Journal of Learning Disabilities, 33*(4).

Manis, F., & Freedman, L. (2001). The relationship of naming speed to multiple reading measures in disabled and normal readers. In M. Wolf (Ed.), *Dyslexia, fluency, and the brain.* Timonium, MD: York Press.

Maricle, D., Johnson, W., & Avirett, E. (2010). Assessing and intervening with children with executive function disorders. In D. Miller (Ed.), *Best practices in school neuropsychology: Guidelines for effective practice, assessment, and evidence-based intervention.* Hoboken, NJ: Wiley.

Maricle, D., Psimas-Fraser, L., Muenke, R., & Miller, D. (2010). Assessing and intervening with children with math disorders. In D. Miller (Ed.), *Best practices in school neuropsychology: Guidelines for effective practice, assessment, and evidence-based intervention.* Hoboken, NJ: Wiley.

Marx, M. H., & Cronan-Hillix, W. A. (1987). *Systems and theories in psychology* (4th ed.). New York: McGraw-Hill.

Mastergeorge, A. M. (2013). Speech and language disorders in childhood: A neurodevelopmental perspective. In R. L. Hansen & S. J. Rogers (Eds.), *Autism and other neurodevelopmental disorders. Washington, DC: American Psychiatric Publishing.*

Matlin, M. (1989). *Cognition* (2nd ed.). Fort Worth, TX: Holt, Rinehart, and Winston.

Matson, J. L., & Nebel-Schwalm, M. S. (2007). Comorbid psychopathology with autism spectrum disorder in children: An overview. *Research in Developmental Disabilities, 28,* 341–352.

Mattson, S., & Vaurio, L. (2010). Fetal alcohol spectrum disorders. In K. Yeates, M. Ris, H. Taylor, & B. Pennington (Eds.), *Pediatric neuropsychology: Research, theory, and practice (2nd ed.). New York: Guilford.*

Mayes, S. D., & Calhoun, S. L. (2003). Ability profiles in children in autism: Influence of age and I.Q. *Autism, 6,* 83–98.

Mayo Clinic. (2014). Rett syndrome. Retrieved from http://www.mayoclinic.org/diseases-conditions/rett-syndrome/basics/symptoms/con-20028086

McIntosh, D., & Decker, S. (2005). Understanding and evaluating special education, IDEA, ADA, NCLB, and Section 504 in school neuropsychology. In R. D'Amato, E. Fletcher-Janzen, & C. Reynolds (Eds.), *Handbook of school neuropsychology.* Hoboken, NJ: Wiley.

Meece, J., & Daniels, D. (2008). *Child and adolescent development for educators* (3rd ed.). Boston: McGraw-Hill.

Meltzer, L. (Ed.) (2007). *Executive function in education: From theory to practice.* New York: Guilford.

Meltzer, L., & Krishnan, K. (2007). Executive function disabilities and learning disabilities. In L. Meltzer (Ed.), *Executive function in education: From theory to practice.* New York: Guilford.

Mervis, C., & John, A. (2010). Intellectual disability syndromes. In K. Yeates, M. Ris, H. Taylor, & B. Pennington (Eds.), *Pediatric neuropsychology: Research, theory, and practice.* New York: Guilford.

Miles, T. R., & Miles, E. (1992). *Dyslexia and mathematics.* New York: Routledge.

Miller, C. A., Kail, R., Leonard, L. B., & Tomblin, J. B. (2001). Speed of processing in children with specific language impairment. *Journal of Speech, Language and Hearing Research, 44*, 416.

Miller, D. (Ed.) (2010a). *Best practices in school neuropsychology: Guidelines for effective practice, assessment, and evidence-based intervention*. Hoboken, NJ: Wiley.

Miller, D. (2010b). School neuropsychology training and credentialing. In D. Miller (Ed.), *Best practices in school neuropsychology: Guidelines for effective practice, assessment, and evidence-based intervention*. Hoboken, NJ: Wiley.

Miller, D., & Defina, P. (2010). The application of neuroscience to the practice of school neuropsychology. In D. Miller (Ed.), *Best practices in school neuropsychology: Guidelines for effective practice, assessment, and evidence-based intervention*. Hoboken, NJ: Wiley.

Miller, J., & Blasik, J. (2010). Assessing and intervening with children with memory and learning disorders. In D. Miller (Ed.), *Best practices in school neuropsychology: Guidelines for effective practice, assessment, and evidence-based intervention*. Hoboken, NJ: Wiley.

Miller, M. (2011). What college teachers should know about memory: A perspective from cognitive psychology. *College Teaching, 59*(3), 117–122.

Minshew, N. J., & Williams, D. L. (2008). Brain-behavior connections in autism. In K. D. Buron & P. Wolfberg (Eds.), *Learners on the autism spectrum: Preparing highly qualified educators*. Shawnee Mission, KS: Autism Asperger.

Mirsky, A. F. (2005). Disorders of attention: A neuropsychological perspective. In G. R. Lyon & N. A Krasnegor (Eds.), *Attention, memory, and executive function*. Baltimore, MD: Paul H. Brookes.

Moats, L. (1998). Reading, spelling, and writing disabilities in the middle grades: Learning. In B. Wong (Ed.), *Learning about learning disabilities*. Orlando, FL: Academic Press.

Moats, L. (2001). Overcoming the language gap: Invest generously in teacher professional development. *American Educator, 25*, 5–7.

Moats, L., & Lyon, G. R. (1996). Wanted: Teachers with knowledge of language. *Topics in Language Disorders, 16*, 73–86.

Mody, M., & Silliman, E. R. (Eds.) (2008a). *Brain, behavior, and learning in language and reading disorders*. New York: Guilford.

Mody, M., & Silliman, E. R. (2008b). The language-reading interface: Associations and dissociations within an atypically developing system. In M. Mody & E. R. Silliman (Eds.), *Brain, behavior, and learning in language and reading disorders*. New York: Guilford.

Mody, M., & Silliman, E. R. (2008c). Learning to read and reading to learn: The interaction among cognitive capacity, linguistic abilities, and the learning environment. In M. Mody & E. R. Silliman (Eds.), *Brain, behavior, and learning in language and reading disorders*. New York: Guilford.

Montague, M., & Jitendra, A. (Eds.) (2006). *Teaching mathematics to middle school students with learning disabilities.* New York: Guilford.

Moore, K. L., & Dalley, A. F. (1999). *Clinically oriented anatomy* (4th ed.). Philadelphia: Lippincott, Williams, and Wilkins.

Mrazik, M., Bender, S., & Makovichuk, C. (2010). Memory functioning in post-secondary students with learning disabilities. *Research in Higher Education Journal, 8,* 1–9.

Myer, M. S., & Felton, R. H. (1999). Repeated reading to enhance fluency: Old approaches and new directions. *Annals of Dyslexia, 49,* 283–306.

Myles, B. S., & Simpson, R. L. (1998). *Asperger syndrome: A guide for educators and parents.* Austin, TX: PRO-ED.

Naidu, S. (1997). Rett syndrome: A disorder affecting early brain growth. *Annals of Neurology, 42,* 3–10.

Nation, K., Marshall, C. M., & Altman, G. T. M. (2003). Investigating individual differences in children's real-time sentence comprehension using language-mediated eye movements. *Journal of Experimental Child Psychology, 86,* 314–330.

National Center for Learning Disabilities. (2014). Checking up on learning disabilities. Retrieved from http://www.ncid.org/types-learning-disabilities/what-is-ld/checking-up-on-learning'disabilities.

National Human Genome Research Institute and National Institutes of Health. (2014). Learning about fragile X syndrome. http://www.genome.gov.

National Institute of Neurological Disorders and Stroke. . (2008a). Autism fact sheet. Retrieved from http://www.ninds.nih.gov/disorders/autism/detail_autism.htm.

National Institute of Neurological Disorders and Stroke. (2008b). Learning disabilities. Retrieved from http://www.ninds.nih.gov/disorders/learningdisabilities/learningdisabilities.htm.

National Joint Committee on Learning Disabilities. (1988). LD Online. Retrieved from http://www.ldonline.org.

National Organization on Fetal Alcohol Syndrome (2014). FASD: What everyone should know. Retrieved from http://www.nofas.org.

National Reading Panel. (2000). *Teaching children to read: An evidence-based assessment of the scientific research literature on reading and its implications for reading instruction.* Washington, DC: National Institute of Child Health and Human Development.

National Tourette Syndrome Association. (2014). What is Tourette syndrome? Retrieved from http://www.tsa-usa.org.

Nicolson, R., & Fawcett, A. (2001). Dyslexia, learning, and the cerebellum. In M. Wolf (Ed.), *Dyslexia, fluency, and the brain.* Timonium, MD: York Press.

Nolte, J. (2009). *The human brain: An introduction to its functional anatomy.* Philadelphia: Mosby Elsevier.

Noterdaeme, M., Amorosa, H., Mildenberger, K., Sitter, S., & Minnow, F. (2001). Evaluation of attention problems in children with autism and children with a specific language disorder. *European Child and Adolescent Psychiatry, 11,* 219–225.

O'Connor, I. M., & Klein, P. D. (2004). Exploration of strategies for facilitating the reading comprehension of high-functioning students with autism spectrum disorders. *Journal of Autism and Developmental Disorders, 34*(2), 115–127.

O'Connor, R. E., & Vadasy, P. F. (Eds.) (2011). *Handbook of reading interventions.* New York: Guilford.

Odom, S., Horner, R., Snell, M., & Blacher, J. (2007). *Handbook of developmental disabilities.* New York: Guilford.

Ojose, B. (2008). Applying Piaget's theory of cognitive development to mathematics instruction. *Mathematics Educator, 18*(1), 26–30.

O'Leary, C., Leonard, H., Bourke, J., D'Antoine, H., Batu, A., & Bower, C. (2013). Intellectual disability: Population-based estimates of the proportion attributable to maternal alcohol use disorder during pregnancy. *Developmental Medicine and Child Neurology,* 55(3), 271–277.

Olson, M., & Hergenhahn, B. R. (2009). *An introduction to theories of learning.* Upper Saddle River, NJ: Pearson/Prentice Hall.

Orasanu, J. (1986). *Reading comprehension: From research to practice.* Hillsdale, NJ: Lawrence Erlbaum.

Ornstein, R., & Thompson, R. F. (1984). *The amazing brain.* Boston: Houghton Mifflin.

Ozonoff, S. (2010). Autism spectrum disorders. In K. Yeates, M. Ris, H. Taylor, & B. Pennington (Eds.), *Pediatric neuropsychology: Research, theory, and practice.* New York: Guilford.

Ozonoff, S., Pennington, B. F., & Rogers, S. J. (1991). Executive function deficits in high-functioning autistic individuals: Relationship to theory of mind. *Journal of Child Psychology and Psychiatry, 32,* 1081–1105.

Palombo, J. (2006). *Nonverbal learning disabilities: A clinical perspective.* New York:Norton.

Papilia, D., & Olds, S. W. (1992). *Human development (5th ed.). New York: McGraw-Hill.*

Pavlidis, G., & Fisher, D. (Eds.) (1987). *Dyslexia: Its neuropsychology and treatment.* New York: Wiley.

Pennington, B. (2009). *Diagnosing learning disorders: A neuropsychological framework* (2nd ed.). New York: Guilford.

Pennington, B. F., & Ozonoff, S. (1996). Executive functions and developmental psychopathologies. *Journal of Child Psychology and Psychiatry, 37,* 51–87.

Percy, A. K. (2002). Rett syndrome: Current status and new vistas. *Neurologic Clinics, 20,* 1125–1141.

Peterson, R., & Pennington, B. (2010). Reading disability. In K. O. Yeates,

M. D. Ris, H. G. Taylor, & B. F. Pennington (Eds.), *Pediatric neuropsychology: Research, theory, and practice.* New York: Guilford.

Piaget, J. (1972). *The psychology of the child.* New York: Basic Books.

Plessen, K. (2013). Tic disorders and Tourette's syndrome. *European Child and Adolescent Psychiatry, 22,* 55–60.

Pressley, M., & McCormick, C. (2007). *Child and adolescent development for educators.* New York: Guilford.

Professional Affairs Board of the British Psychological Society. (2000). *Learning disabilities: Definitions and contexts.* Leicester, UK: British Psychological Society.

Pueschel, S. M. (1992). Phenotype characteristics. In S. M. Pueschel & J. K. Pueschel (Eds.), *Biomedical concerns in persons with Down syndrome.* Baltimore, MD: Brookes.

Quinn, M. (2010). Assessing and intervening with children with speech and language disorders. In D. Miller (Ed.), *Best practices in school neuropsychology: Guidelines for effective practice, assessment, and evidence-based intervention.* Hoboken, NJ: Wiley.

Rayner, K., & Pollatsek, A. (1989). *The psychology of reading.* New York: Prentice-Hall.

Reid, G. (2003). *Dyslexia: A practitioner's handbook* (3rd ed.). Hoboken, NJ: Wiley.

Reynolds, C., & French, C. (2005). The brain as a dynamic organ of information processing and learning. In R. D'Amato, E. Fletcher-Janzen, & C. Reynolds (Eds.), *Handbook of school neuropsychology.* Hoboken, NJ: Wiley.

Reynolds, C., & Mayfield, J. (2011). Neuropsychological assessment in genetically linked neurodevelopmental disorders. In S. Goldstein & C. Reynolds (Eds.), *Handbook of neurodevelopmental and genetic disorders in children* (2nd ed.). New York: Guilford.

Riccio, C., & Pizzitola-Jarratt, K. (2005). Abnormalities of neurological development. In R. D'Amato, E. Fletcher-Janzen, & C. Reynolds (Eds.), *Handbook of school neuropsychology.* Hoboken, NJ: Wiley.

Ripley, K. (2001). *Inclusion for children with dyspraxia/DCD: A handbook for teachers.* New York: Taylor and Francis.

Robertson, M. M. (2006). Attention deficit hyperactivity disorder, tics, and Tourette's syndrome: The relationship and treatment implications. A commentary. *Child and Adolescent Psychiatry, 15*(1), 1–11.

Roessner, P. J. (2011). Tourette's disorder and other tic disorders in *DSM-5:* A comment. *European Child and Adolescent Psychiatry, 20*(2), 71–74.

Rogers, S., Ozonoff, S., & Hanson, R. (2013). Autism spectrum disorders. In R. Hanson & S. Rogers (Eds.), *Autism and other neurodevelopmental disorders.* Arlington, VA: American Psychiatric Publishing.

Rondal, J. A., Hodapp, R. M., Soresi, S., Dykens, E. M., & Nota, L. (2004). *Intellectual disabilities: Genetics, behavior and inclusion.* London: Whurr.

Rourke, B. (1989). *Nonverbal learning disabilities: The syndrome and the model*. New York: Guilford.

Rourke, B. (1995a). The NLD syndrome and the white matter model. In *Syndrome of nonverbal learning disabilities: Neurodevelopmental manifestations*. New York: Guilford.

Rourke, B. (Ed.) (1995b). *Syndrome of nonverbal learning disabilities: Neurodevelopmental manifestations*. New York: Guilford.

Rourke, B., Bakker, D., Fisk, J., & Strang, J. (1983). *Child neuropsychology: An introduction to theory, research, and practice*. New York: Guilford.

Rourke, B., & Conway, J. (1997). Disabilities of arithmetic and mathematical reasoning: Perspective from neurology and neuropsychology. *Journal of Learning Disabilities, 30*(1), 34–46.

Rourke, B., & Fuerts, D. (1991). *Learning disabilities and psychosocial functioning*. New York: Guilford.

Roth, I., & Frisby, J. P. (1986). *Perception and representation: A cognitive approach*. Philadelphia: Open University Press.

Ruhl, K. L., Hughes, C. A., & Camarata, S. T. (1992). Analysis of the expressive and receptive language characteristics of emotionally handicapped students served in public school settings. *Journal of Childhood Communication Disorders, 13*, 165–176.

Rumelhart, D. E., & Norman, D. A. (1983). Representation in memory. In R. C. Atkinson, R. J. Herrnstein, G. Lindzey, and R. D. Luce (Eds), *Handbook of experimental psychology*. New York: Wiley.

Rypma, B., & D'Esposito, M. (2000). Isolating the neural mechanisms of age-related changes in human working memory. *Nature Neuroscience, 3*(5),509–515.

Sadock, B. J., & Sadock, V. A. (2003). *Synopsis of psychiatry: Behavioral sciences/clinical psychiatry* (9th ed.). Philadelphia: Lippincott Williams and Wilkins.

Sanders, M. (2001). *Understanding dyslexia and the reading process: A guide for educators and parents*. Boston: Allyn and Bacon.

Sattler, J. M. (2001). *Assessment of children: Cognitive applications* (4th ed.). San Diego, CA: Jerome M. Sattler.

Schachter, J. (1999). *Reading programs that work: A review of programs for pre-kindergarten to 4th grade*. Santa Monica, CA: Milken Family Foundation.

Schalock, R. L. (2009). *Intellectual disability: Definition, classification, and system of supports* (11th ed.). Washington, DC: American Association on Intellectual and Developmental Disabilities.

Schank, R. (1982). *Reading and understanding: Teaching from the perspective of artificial intelligence*. Mahwah, NJ: Lawrence Erlbaum.

Schmitt, M. B., Justice, L. M., & Pentimonti, J. M. (2013). Language processes: Characterization and prevention of language-learning disabilities. In H. L. Swanson, K. R. Harris, & S. Graham (Eds.), *Handbook of learning disabilities* (2nd ed.). New York: Guilford.

Schultz, D. P., & Schultz, S. E. (2008). *A history of modern psychology* (9th ed.). Belmont, CA: Wadsworth.

Schweitzer, J. B., Pakyurek, M., & Dixon, J. F. (2013). Attention deficit/ hyperactivity disorder: Signs, symptoms, and developmental course. In R. Hanson & S. Rogers (Eds.), *Autism and other neurodevelopmental disorders*. Arlington, VA: American Psychiatric Publishing.

Seligman, L. (2006). *Theories of counseling and psychotherapy: Systems, strategies, and skills* (2nd ed.). Upper Saddle River, NJ: Prentice-Hall.

Semrud-Clikeman, M., Fine, J. G., & Harder, L. (2005). Providing neuropsychological services to students with learning disabilities. In R. D'Amato, E. Fletcher-Janzen, & C. Reynolds (Eds.), *Handbook of school neuropsychology*. Hoboken, NJ: Wiley.

Shaffer, D., & Kipp, K. (2009). *Developmental psychology: Childhood and adolescence*. Belmont, CA: Wadsworth.

Shah, N. S., & Donald, A. G. (1986). *Movement disorders*. New York: Plenum.

Shankweiler, D., & Liberman, I. Y. (1972). Language by eye and by ear. In J. F. Kavanaugh & I. Y. Liberman (Eds.), *Misreading: A search for causes* (pp. 293–317). Cambridge, MA: MIT Press.

Shaywitz, S. (2003). *Overcoming dyslexia: A new and complete science-based program for reading problems at any level*. New York: Knopf.

Simonoff, E., Pickles, A., Charman, T., Chandler, S., Loucas, T., & Baird, G. (2008). Psychiatric disorders in children with autism spectrum disorders: Prevalence, comorbidity, and associated factors in a population-derived sample. *Journal of American Academy of Child and Adolescent Psychiatry, 47,* 921–929.

Singer, M. (1990). *Psychology of language: An introduction to sentence and discourse processes*. Hillsdale, NJ: Lawrence Erlbaum.

Snowling, M. (2001). *Dyslexia*. Oxford: Blackwell.

Snowling, M., & Hayiou-Thomas, M. (2010). Specific language impairment. In K. Yeates, M. Ris, H. Taylor, & B. Pennington (Eds.), *Pediatric neuropsychology: Research, theory, and practice*. New York: Guilford.

Sousa, D. (2001). *How the brain learns*. Thousand Oaks, CA: Corwin.

Sousa, D. (2008a). *How the brain learns mathematics*. Thousand Oaks, CA: Corwin.

Sousa, D. (2008b). *How the special needs brain learns* (2nd ed.). Thousand Oaks, CA: Corwin.

Spafford, C., & Grosser, G. (1996). *Dyslexia: Research and resource guide*. Boston: Allyn and Bacon.

Spear, L. (2010). *The behavioral neuroscience of adolescence*. New York: Norton.

Spreen, O., Risser, A., & Edgell, D. (1995). *Developmental neuropsychology.* Oxford: Oxford University Press.

Spreen, O., & Strauss, E. (1998). *A compendium of neuropsychological tests: Administration, norms, and commentary* (2nd ed.). New York: Oxford University Press.

Sprinthall, N., & Sprinthall, R. (1990). *Educational psychology: A developmental approach* (5th ed.). New York: McGraw-Hill.

Squire, L. R., & Zola, S. M. (2000). Episodic memory, semantic memory, and amnesia. In M. S. Gazzaniga (Ed.), *Cognitive neuroscience: A reader.* Oxford: Blackwell.

Stacey, R. (2003). *Thinking about language: Helping students say what they mean and mean what they say.* Prides Crossing, MA: Landmark School.

Stanovich, K. (1986). Matthew effects in reading: Some consequences of individual differences in acquisition of literacy. *Reading Research Quarterly, 4,* 360–407.

Stanovich, K. (1988). The dyslexic and garden variety poor reader: The phonological-core variable-difference model. *Journal of Learning Disabilities, 21,* 590–604.

Stanovich, K. E. (1992). Speculations on the causes and consequences of individual differences in early reading acquisition. In P. B. Gough, L. C. Ehri, & R. Treiman (Eds.), *Reading acquisition* (pp. 307–342). Mahwah, NJ: Lawrence Erlbaum.

Stein, J. (2001). The neurobiology of reading difficulties. In M. Wolf (Ed.), *Dyslexia, fluency, and the brain.* Timonium, MD: York Press.

Sternberg, R. J. (1986). *Intelligence applied: Understanding and increasing your intellectual skills.* New York: Harcourt Brace Jovanovich.

Sternberg, R. J., & Berg, C. A. (1986). Quantitative integration: Definitions of intelligence: A comparison of the 1921 and 1986 symposia. In R. J. Sternberg & D. K. Detterman (Eds.), *What is intelligence?* (pp. 155–162). Norwood, NJ: Ablex.

Stone, C. A., Silliman, E. R., Ehren, B. J., & Wallach, G. P. (2014). *Handbook of language and literacy: Development and disorders.* New York: Guilford.

Storch, E. A. (2009). Sleep-related problems in youth with Tourette's syndrome and chronic tic disorder. *Child and Adolescent Mental Health, 14(2),* 97–103.

Straube, B. (2012, July 24). An overview of neuro-cognitive processes involved in the encoding, consolidation, and retrieval of true and false memories. *Behavioral and Brain Functions, 8,* 35.

Suchy, Y. (2011). *Clinical psychology of emotion.* New York: Guilford.

Sugden, D., & Chambers, M. (Eds.) (2005). *Children with developmental coordination disorder.* Hoboken, NJ: Wiley.

Swanson, H. L. (2009). What are the most important instructional ingredients for successful reading comprehension programs for students with learning disabilities? In G. Sideridis & T. A. Citro (Eds.), *Strategies in reading for struggling learners*. Weston, MA: Learning Disabilities Worldwide.

Swanson, H., Cochran, K., & Eivers, C. (1990). Can learning disabilities be determined from working memory performance? *Journal of Learning Disabilities, 23*, 59–67.

Swanson, H. L., Harris, K. R., & Graham, S. (2013). *Handbook of learning disabilities* (2nd ed.). New York: Guilford.

Tager-Flusberg, H., & Anderson, M. (1991). The development of contingent discourse ability in autistic children. *Journal of Child Psychology and Psychiatry, 32*, 1123–1134.

Teale, W. H. (1995). Young children and reading: Trends across the twentieth century. *Journal of Education, 177*, 95–127.

Teeter, P. A., & Semrud-Clikeman, M. (2007). *Child neuropsychology: Assessment and interventions for neurodevelopmental disorders*. Boston: Allyn and Bacon.

Teeter-Ellison, P. A. (2005). School neuropsychology and attention deficit/hyperactivity disorder. In R. D'Amato, E. Fletcher-Janzen, & C. Reynolds (Eds.), *Handbook of school neuropsychology*. Hoboken, NJ: Wiley.

Terman, L. M. (1921). A symposium: Intelligence and its measurement. *Journal of Educational Psychology, 12*, 127–133.

Termine, C., Stella, G., Capsoni, C., Rosso, E., Binda, A., Pirola, A., et al. (2007). Neuropsychological profile of pre-schoolers with metaphonological difficulties: Results from a non-clinical sample. *Child: Care, Health and Development, 33*, 703–712.

Tofallo, D. (2010). Linking school neuropsychology with response-to-intervention models. In D. Miller (Ed.), *Best practices in school neuropsychology: Guidelines for effective practice, assessment, and evidence-based intervention*. Hoboken, NJ: Wiley.

Torgeson, J. (1988). Studies of children with learning disabilities who perform poorly on memory span tasks. *Journal of Learning Disabilities, 21*, 605–612.

Torgeson, J., & Houck, G. (1990). Processing deficiencies of learning disabled children who perform poorly on the Digit Span subtest. *Journal of Educational Psychology, 72*, 141–160.

Torgeson, J., Rashotte, C., & Alexander, A. (2001). Principles of fluency instruction in reading: Relationships with established empirical outcomes. In M. Wolf (Ed.), *Dyslexia, fluency and the brain*. Timonium, MD: York Press.

Torgeson, J. K., Wagner, R. K., & Rashotte, C. A. (1994). Longitudinal studies of phonological processing and reading. *Journal of Learning Disabilities, 27*, 276–286.

Torgeson, J. K., Wagner, R. K., Rashotte, C. A., & Hecht, S. (1997). Contributions of phonological awareness and rapid automatic naming ability to the growth of word-reading skills in second- to fifth-grade children. *Scientific Studies of Reading, 1*(2), 161–195.

Tovi, A., Buterbaugh, A., Love, K., & Visootsak, J. (2013). A male with concurrence of Down syndrome and fragile X syndrome. *Case Reports in Genetics, 1–4.*

Trautman, R., Gidden, J., & Jurs, S. (1990). Language risk factors in emotionally disturbed children within a school and day treatment program. *Journal of Childhood Communication Disorders, 13,* 123–133.

Tuchman, R. (2011). Epilepsy and encephalography in autism spectrum disorder. In D. G. Amaral, G. Dawson, & D. Geschwind (Eds.). *Autism spectrum disorders.* New York: Oxford University Press.

Tupper, D. E., & Sondell, S. K. (2004). Motor disorders and neuropsychological development: A historical appreciation. In D. Dewey & D. E. Tupper (Eds.), *Developmental motor disorders: A neuropsychological perspective.* New York: Guilford.

United Kingdom Department of Health. (2014). Learning disabilities. Retrieved from http://www.gov.uk/learning-disabilities-program-board.

Van Acker, R. (1991). Rett syndrome: A review of current knowledge. *Journal of Autism and Developmental Disabilities, 21,* 381–406.

Vargo, F. E. (1992). *Wechsler subtest profiles: Diagnostic usefulness with dyslexic children* (Unpublished doctoral dissertation). American International College, Springfield, MA.

Vargo, F. E. (2007). *Diagnosis and remediation of early reading problems in young children: A neurodevelopmentally based integrated program* (Unpublished master's thesis). Union Institute and University, Cincinnati, OH.

Vargo, F. E. (2008). Counseling considerations and implications for individuals with language disabilities. In N. Young & C. Michaels (Eds.), *Counseling in a complex society.* Amherst, MA: Practitioner Publications/Psychosynthesis Center Press.

Vargo, F. E., Grosser, G., & Spafford, C. (1995). Digit Span and other WISC-R scores in the diagnosis of dyslexia in children. *Perceptual and Motor Skills, 80,* 219–229.

Vargo, F. E., Judah, R. D., & Young, N. D. (2010). Executive function disorders and learning disabilities: The connection, diagnosis, and strategies for intervention . In N. G. Wamba & T. A. Citro (Eds.), *Learning differences: Research, practice, and advocacy.* Weston, MA: Learning Disabilities Worldwide.

Vargo, F. E., & Young, N. (2011a). What are learning disabilities? Learning Disabilities Worldwide.

Vargo, F. E., & Young, N. (2011b). What are the signs of a learning disability? Learning Disabilities Worldwide. Retrieved from http://www.ldworldwide.org/what-are-the-signs-of-ld.

Vargo, F. E., Young, N., & Judah, R. (2008). The role of word automaticity and reading fluency in reading disorders: A guide for assessment, diagnosis, and remediation. In *Insights on learning disabilities: From prevailing theories to validated practices.* Weston, MA: Learning Disabilities Worldwide.

Vargo, F. E., Young, N., & Vargo, C. P. (2004). The role of phonological processing in reading disorders: A guide for assessment, diagnosis, and remediation. *Journal of the Learning Disabilities Association of Massachusetts, 15*(1).

Vaughn, S., Swanson, E., & Solis, M. (2013). Reading comprehension for adolescents with significant reading problems. In H. L. Swanson, K. R. Harris, & S. Graham (Eds.), *Handbook of learning disabilities* (2nd ed.). New York: Guilford.

Vellutino, F., & Scanlon, P. (1987). Phonological coding, phonological awareness, and reading ability: Evidence from a longitudinal and experimental study. *Merrill Palmer Quarterly, 33,* 321–363.

Wade, M. G., Johnson, D., & Mally, K. (2005). DCD and overlapping conditions. In D. Sugden & M. Chambers (Eds.), *Children with developmental coordination disorder.* London: Whurr.

Wadlington, E., & Wadlington, P. L. (2008). Helping students with mathematical disabilities to succeed. *Preventing School Failure,53*(1), 2–7.

Wagner, R. K., & Torgesen, J. K. (1987). The nature of phonological processing and its causal role in the acquisition of reading skills. *Psychological Bulletin, 101,* 192–212.

Wagner, R., Torgesen, J., & Rashotte, C. (1999). *The comprehensive test of phonological processing: Examiner's manual.* San Antonio, TX: Pearson Assessments.

Wallach, G. P., Charlton, S., & Bartholomew, J. C. (2014). The spoken-written comprehension connection: Constructive intervention strategies. In C. A. Stone, E. R. Silliman, B. J. Ehren, & G. P. Wallach (Eds.), *Handbook of language and literacy: Development and disorders.* New York: Guilford.

Walsh, R., de Bie, R., & Fox, S. H. (2013). *Movement disorders.* New York: Oxford University Press.

Wang, L. W., Tancredi, D. J., & Thomas, D. W. (2011). The prevalence of gastrointestinal problems in children across the United States with autism spectrum disorders from families with multiple affected members. *Journal of Developmental and Behavioral Pediatrics, 32,* 351–360.

Wechsler, D. (1958). *The measurement and appraisal of adult intelligence* (4th ed.). Baltimore, MD: Williams and Wilkins.

Wechsler, D. (2001). *Wechsler intelligence scale for children–fourth edition: Administration and scoring manual.* San Antonio, TX: Harcourt Assessment.

Wechsler, D. (2002). *Wechsler preschool and primary scale of intelligence: Administration and scoring manual.* San Antonio, TX: Harcourt Assessment.

Weismer, S. E., Plante, E., Jones, M., & Tamblin, J. B. (2005). A functional magnetic resonance imaging investigation of verbal working memory in adolescents with specific language impairment. *Journal of Speech, Language and Hearing Research, 48*, 405–425.

Westby, C. E. (2014). A language perspective on executive functioning, metacognition, and self-regulation in reading. In C. A. Stone, E. R. Silliman, B. J. Ehren, & G. P. Wallach (Eds.), *Handbook of language and literacy: Development and disorders.* New York: Guilford.

Westby, C. E., & Cutler, S. K. (1994). Language and ADHD: Understanding the bases and treatment of self-regulatory deficits. *Topics in Language Disorders, 14*, 58–67.

Weyandt, L. (2005). Executive function in children, adolescents, and adults with attention deficit disorder. *Developmental Neuropsychology, 27*(1).

Whitaker, S. (2013). *Intellectual disability: An inability to cope with an intellectually demanding world.* New York: Palgrave Macmillan.

White, S. W., Oswald, D., Ollendick, T., & Scahill, L. (2009). Anxiety in children and adolescents with autism spectrum disorder. *Clinical Psychology Review, 29*, 216–229.

Wickelgren, W. A. (1981). Human learning and memory. *Annual Review of Psychology,32*(1),21–52.

Wiig, E., Zureich, P., & Chan, H. (2000). A clinical rationale for assessing rapid automatized naming in children with language disorders. *Journal of Learning Disabilities,33*(4).

Willcutt, E. (2010). Attention deficithyperactivity disorder. In K. Yeates, M. Ris, H. Taylor, & B. Pennington (Eds.), *Pediatric neuropsychology: Research, theory, and practice.* New York: Guilford.

Willis, W. G. (2005). Foundations of developmental neuroanatomy. In R. D'Amato, E. Fletcher-Janzen, & C. Reynolds (Eds.), *Handbook of school neuropsychology.* Hoboken, NJ: Wiley.

Wilmhurst, L. (2009). *Abnormal child psychology.* New York: Routledge.

Windsor, J., & Kohnert, K. (2008). Processing measures of cognitive-linguistic interactions for children with language impairment and reading disabilities. In M. Mody & E. R. Silliman (Eds.), *Brain, behavior, and learning in language and reading disorders.* New York: Guilford.

Wishaw, I., & Kolb, B. (2008). *Fundamentals of human neuropsychology.* New York: Worth.

Wolf, M. (1991). Naming speed and reading: The contribution of the cognitive neurosciences. *Reading and Research Quarterly, 26*, 123–141.

Wolf, M. (Ed.) (2001). *Dyslexia, fluency, and the Brain.* Timonium, MD: York Press.

Wolf, M. (2007). *Proust and the squid: The story and science of the reading brain.* New York: Harper.

Wolf, M., & Bowers, P. (1999). The double-deficit hypothesis for the developmental dyslexias. *Journal of Educational Psychology, 91*(3), 415–438.

Wolf, M., Bowers, P., & Biddle, K. (2000). Naming-speed processes, timing, and reading: A conceptual review. *Journal of Learning Disabilities,33*(4).

Wolf, M., & Katzir-Cohen, T. (2001). Reading fluency and its intervention. *Scientific Studies of Reading, 5*(3), 211–239.

Wolf-Schein, E. G. (1992). On the association between fragile X chromosome, mental handicap, and autistic disorder. *Developmental Disabilities Bulletin, 20, 13–30.*

Woods, D., & Miltenberger, R. (2009). *Tic disorders, trichotillomania, and other repetitive behavior disorders: Behavioral approaches to analysis and treatment.* New York: Springer.

World Health Organization. (2014). Retrieved from http://www.who.int.

Yalof, J., & McGrath, M. C. (2010). Assessing and intervening with nonverbal learning disabilities. In D. Miller (Ed.), *Best practices in school neuropsychology: Guidelines for effective practice, assessment, and evidence-based intervention.* Hoboken, NJ: Wiley.

Yeager, M., & Yeager, D. (2013). *Executive function and child development.* New York: Norton.

Yeates, K., Ris, M., Taylor, H., & Pennington, B. (2010). *Pediatric neuropsychology: Research, theory, and practice* (2nd ed.). New York: Guilford.

Yeo, D. (2005). *Dyslexia, dyspraxia, and mathematics.* Hoboken, NJ: Wiley.

Zemelman, S., Daniels, H., & Hyde, A. (2005). *Best practice: Today's standards for teaching and learning in America's schools.* Portsmouth, NH: Heinemann.

Index